The ACCP Field Guide to Becoming a Standout
Pharmacy Residency Candidate

PROPERTY OF
WUSOP

# The ACCP Field Guide to Becoming a Standout Pharmacy Residency Candidate

Jerry L. Bauman, Pharm.D., FCCP, FACC, Executive Editor
Keri A. Sims, Pharm.D., BCPS, Associate Editor

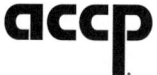

American College of Clinical Pharmacy
Lenexa, Kansas

Director of Professional Development: Nancy M. Perrin, M.A., CAE
Associate Director of Professional Development: Wafa Dahdal, Pharm.D., BCPS (AQ Cardiology)
Publications Project Manager: Janel Mosley
Desktop Publisher/Graphic Designer: Jen DeYoe, B.F.A.
Medical Editor: Kimma Sheldon, Ph.D., M.A.

For order information or questions contact:
American College of Clinical Pharmacy
13000 West 87th Street Parkway, Suite 100
Lenexa, Kansas 66215
(913) 492-3311
(913) 492-0088 (Fax)
accp@accp.com

Copyright © 2012 by the American College of Clinical Pharmacy. No part of this publication may be reproduced, stored in a retrieval system, or transmitted, in any form or by any means, electronic or mechanical, including photocopy, without prior written permission of the American College of Clinical Pharmacy.

Printed in the United States of America
ISBN: 978-1-932658-90-3
Library of Congress Control Number: 2012951819

# TABLE OF CONTENTS

Introduction ........................................................................................... vii
*Jerry L. Bauman, Pharm.D., FCCP, FACC*

Step I: Define and Redefine Your Goals ............................................. 1
*Stuart T. Haines, Pharm.D., FCCP, BCPS, BCACP*

Step II: Making the Grade ................................................................... 27
*Dana P. Hammer, R.Ph., M.S., Ph.D.*

Step III: Get Involved .......................................................................... 41
*Janet P. Engle, Pharm.D., FAPhA*

Step IV: Develop Leadership and Management Abilities ............... 57
*Donald E. Letendre, Pharm.D.*
*Brandon J. Patterson, Pharm.D.*

Step V: Gain Valuable Work Experience ........................................... 75
*Stephen F. Eckel, Pharm.D., MHA, BCPS*

Step VI: Maximize Experiential Education ....................................... 89
*Brian L. Erstad, Pharm.D., FCCP, BCPS*
*Marcella Hoyland, Pharm.D., BCPS*

Step VII: Expand Your Network ......................................................... 113
*Keri A. Sims, Pharm.D., BCPS*

Step VIII: Engage in Research and Scholarship ............................... 129
*Jerry L. Bauman, Pharm.D., FCCP, FACC*

Step IX: Document It All ..................................................................... 149
*Garrett E. Schramm, Pharm.D., BCPS*
*Heather A. Personett, Pharm.D., BCPS*
*Erin M. Nystrom, Pharm.D., BCNSP*

Step X: Step Up to the Plate: Bringing It
Home in Your Final Professional Year ............................................. 167
*Beth Bryles Phillips, Pharm.D., FCCP, BCPS*

List of Contributors ............................................................................ 195
List of Reviewers ................................................................................. 197
Index ..................................................................................................... 199
Disclosure of Potential Conflicts of Interest .................................... 207

# INTRODUCTION

Jerry L. Bauman, Pharm.D., FCCP, FACC

If you are a Pharm.D. student and are reading this, then you are seriously considering residency training after you graduate. I personally agree with your decision—in fact, I recommend that all Pharm.D. students consider residency training. Why? Simply put, a pharmacy residency is a learning experience that will transform you into a confident, competent, and independent practitioner. In other words, you will become a better pharmacist in an efficient and relatively short time. Although you may think making the decision to do a residency is difficult right now, you will never regret it. In particular, if you want to become a clinical pharmacist, it is almost a prerequisite these days. Frankly, you are not capable of being a truly expert clinical pharmacist when you graduate from pharmacy school, nor are you the so-called "drug expert" (despite what some of your instructors may tell you). And why should anyone expect you to be? Certainly, medical students require post-M.D. internships, residencies, and sometimes fellowships to be truly capable in areas of medicine. Why should this not be true for Pharm.D. students, too? Not all deans would agree with this point of view, but trust me; I was a relatively successful clinical pharmacist for more than 20 years. And the fact is, residency training for pharmacists is the rule rather than the exception in the future of our profession. Both the American College of Clinical Pharmacy and the American Society of Health-System Pharmacists have adopted policies stating that residency training should be a prerequisite for pharmacists engaged in direct patient care by 2020. I personally agree with the ACCP policy.

I did two residencies: one before obtaining my Pharm.D. degree and one afterward. How did they shape my subsequent career? I entered the first one at the University of Illinois Hospital in Chicago with a B.S. degree in pharmacy. Richard Hutchinson, then head of pharmacy practice and director of hospital pharmacy (and who initiated and led the clinical pharmacy program here for 25 years) at the University of Illinois in Chicago (UIC), gave me a surprising chance and accepted me into the residency program. I was the first—and last—B.S. pharmacist he accepted in that residency program—which rather tells you how I did (not well). Lacking a Pharm.D. education and being among coresidents with Pharm.D. degrees, I found that my clinical deficiencies became immediately clear, at least to me (and probably to others). But I profited immensely from the experience, in addition to improving my skills and knowledge, in several important ways. (1) It cemented my passion for clinical pharmacy practice—finally, I knew what I wanted to do in life. (2) It created many important professional mentoring relationships, including one with Dr. Hutchinson, my future boss. (3) It made me realize I needed to get a Pharm.D. degree if I was to seriously pursue my newfound passion. My second residency was at Truman Medical Center after I completed my Pharm.D. degree at the University of Missouri–Kansas City. This incredibly intense (some would say brutal) combined program was led by some of the original clinical pharmacists in the nation, including Kim Kelly, Joel Covinsky, and Bob Elenbaas (all past presidents of ACCP). Now, I could actually apply the foundation of an exceptional Pharm.D. education during my subsequent residency (a much preferred sequence, instead of doing the residency *before* obtaining a Pharm.D. degree). During this second residency, I really gained confidence in clinical situations. It transformed me into a capable clinical pharmacist. In addition, I developed and honed teaching and research skills. Like at the residency at UIC, I was fortunate to develop close mentors who influenced me and helped me throughout my career, and I developed an intense interest in cardiovascular therapeutics, especially the treatment of arrhythmias. So returning to the original question—how did these residencies shape my career? Looking back now—they were **crucial** in almost every aspect! My experience is one reason I tell every student at the UIC College of Pharmacy to consider a residency.

And so can a residency be equally important in your career. Slight problem, however—there aren't enough residencies to go around. In 2012, of the 3,706 PGY1 applicants, 39% did not match with a residency program (similar statistics in 2011). The number of applicants continues to grow faster than the number of residency positions. So apparently, you're not the only one reading this book. At least for now, you must be prepared and have a plan to successfully secure a residency position. You must *distinguish yourself* in some way that makes you stand above the crowd. And that is the purpose of this book: to prepare you to gain acceptance into the residency of your choice. Our approach is organized in a stepwise fashion—from step I (defining your career goals) through step X (the application and interview process). The authors are experts in the field—residency program directors of highly regarded programs, department heads, and deans, all with extensive experience leading programs, evaluating resident candidates, and teaching residents. Each chapter is designed to give you the tools and advice needed to distinguish yourself as an outstanding residency candidate. All are important facets—your grade point average, networking and finding mentors (references), maximizing your experiences during pharmacy school (experiential education, scholarship), and presenting yourself both on paper and in person—and all are necessary to secure the residency of your choice. I should note that the steps do not necessarily follow one another. Rather, as your pharmacy education progresses, the residency application process unfolds, and your perspectives mature, you can refer back to each chapter as required. One additional and crucial ingredient is necessary to using this book: the advice given herein must be combined with your passion for pursuing the career of your choice. Of course, your career path may meander depending on opportunities that arise. A residency is a step in that lifelong journey; if you are passionate about this step, then this book should guide you—and help you emerge from the crowd.

The ACCP Field Guide to Becoming a Standout
Pharmacy Residency Candidate

# STEP I
# DEFINE AND REDEFINE YOUR GOALS

Stuart T. Haines, Pharm.D., FCCP, BCPS, BCACP

**ABBREVIATION IN THIS CHAPTER**

SMART        Specific, measurable, attainable, relevant, and time-bound

> *Knowing yourself is the beginning of all wisdom.*
>
> —Aristotle, ancient Greek philosopher

You may be reading this book because you already have a vision of your future. Perhaps you envision a career in a small, rural community pharmacy providing medication therapy management services to patients. Or, maybe you see yourself leading teaching rounds at a large academic health science center with a crowd of health professional students gathered around as you travel from bedside to bedside. Possibly, you foresee a time when you'll be leading a successful business, providing innovative clinical services using telehealth technologies. But, if you are like most students, you may not (yet) have a clear professional vision. Indeed, you may be struggling to figure out what you want to do after you've earned your degree, perhaps wondering if pharmacy is "right" for you or even second-guessing your past decisions. Here's the good news. We all go through periods of self-doubt. Most of us have only vague notions of what our future will be like, and it rarely materializes exactly how we imagined. This chapter is intended to help you uncover your strengths, find your passions, articulate your personal mission, create a plan to achieve your goals ... while simultaneously preparing you to change course and be flexible.

## ASSESSING YOUR STRENGTHS AND DEVELOPING SELF-KNOWLEDGE

All of us have a unique combination of skills and talents that predisposes us to do well at certain types of work. Skills and talents are a product of both innate aptitude and learned behavior. Although having some innate capacity is helpful, it is only through formal learning and repeated practice that we are able to fully develop our skills and talents. For example, great basketball stars or chess grandmasters are born with innate qualities that predispose them to do well in their fields of expertise. Most great basketball players are taller than average. And most chess grandmasters have better-than-average logico-sequential intelligence. Although these individuals may have been born with these qualities, their exceptional skills and talents came to fruition only through formal instruction (coaching and encouragement) and tons of practice. We'll explore the importance of mindset a little later in this chapter.

Using our skills and talents in constructive ways often gives us a sense of accomplishment. For example, I'm pretty good at being organized, creating schema and structures, and then placing things in them. I use this skill in several ways. I'm able to efficiently construct outlines for presentations and book chapters. I have a penchant for file management, not only physical files but also my digital files; therefore, I can quickly retrieve documents, photos, and Web links. I'm also good at organizing an efficient workflow for both groups and for myself. And my closets, well, let's just say everything has its place. After I've successfully organized my thoughts, my things, and my work or helped others do so, I almost always feel I've achieved something good, useful. Over time, I've honed these skills, through personal experience and reading, to the point that some might say I have a talent for it. The difference between a skill and a talent is a matter of consistency and durability. A talent is a skill that we do well, almost all of the time, in a variety of circumstances.

A passion is something for which we have boundless enthusiasm. We can be passionate about a field of knowledge (e.g., astronomy), a sport (e.g., ice hockey), a pastime (e.g., reading novels), a person (e.g., spouse), objects (e.g., shoes), artistic expression (e.g., jazz music), food (e.g., Mediterranean cuisine), personal finance (e.g., stock trading), or power (e.g., political influence), to name a few. Most of us have more than one passion, but the number of things we can be truly passionate about is probably limited. When we are passionate about something, we like to spend time doing it or being near it. We like to read and talk about it. We buy magazines, watch YouTube videos, and take courses about it. We find ways to connect our passion to other things that, out of necessity, we need to do (e.g., listening to our favorite music while riding the bus). When we engage in our passion, our energy level and emotions improve. Conversely, when we engage in activities we dislike, our spirits and, eventually, our physical health decline.

One of the keys to a successful career is finding the zone where your skills and talents align with your passions and the needs of others (see Figure 1). Where the intersection between our talents and skills meets the needs of others, there are opportunities to earn money. If our passions join our talents and skills, we can achieve excellence. And where all three elements converge, we can find our vocation, a calling in life through which we can make our greatest contributions. Of course, our passions don't always overlap with our skills and talents or with the needs of others. Indeed, many of the things I'm passionate about don't have much value to others. I enjoy a good glass of wine. Most people aren't willing to pay me to drink good wine. I suppose I could pursue a career as a master sommelier or wine steward at some fancy restaurant, but I'm more interested in drinking the wine than in helping others select it. I'm good at organizing, and others value my talent in this area; however, I'm not passionate about it. Admittedly, I didn't discover my vocation while I was in pharmacy school. After working as a pharmacist in a community pharmacy for several years, I discovered

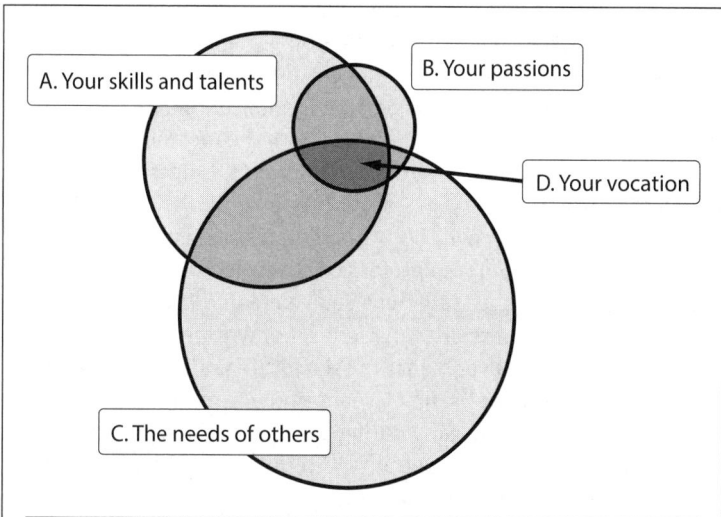

**Figure 1.** A fulfilling career is built around your skills and talents, your passions, and the needs of others. Your vocation is where all three overlap.

that what I loved most about pharmacy practice was the opportunity to coach students and residents, interact directly with patients, and help people use medication wisely. I've grown to understand that teaching, empowering people through education, is my vocation.

*Let yourself be silently drawn by the stronger pull of what you really love.*
—Rumi, thirteenth—century Sufi mystic

Some people are lucky enough to intrinsically know their calling in life at a very early age. But for most of us, it's a journey. Hopefully, you were drawn to pharmacy school because you felt you had some skills and talents that matched well with those required by pharmacists. The admissions committee at your school obviously saw something in you and believed you had the aptitude to navigate a rigorous curriculum. But pharmacy is a very diverse field, and successfully determining your vocation within the profession will help you achieve the most satisfying life possible. So how do you uncover your vocation? Box 1 explains.

Now comes the hard part. After you have taken stock of your talents, skills, and passions and translated them into a potential vocation, it's time to write a personal mission statement. There is no right or wrong way to write a personal mission statement. The intent is to give you some clarity about what gives you a sense of purpose and how you plan to use your talents in a constructive way. Box 2 provides a few pointers on how to develop a personal mission statement. This statement can be as short as a five-word sentence; in that case, you might call it your personal motto. Most mission statements contain a series of brief declarations about the things you care about the most and the ways in which you plan to make a difference in the world. Unless you are a particularly gifted writer, your initial drafts probably won't ring true for you; the words just won't convey your thoughts as precisely as you want. Moreover, at this point in your professional development, you might not be entirely sure that the statement you've created is really "right" for you. That's OK. Your mission statement is not written in stone. Indeed, you should revisit your personal mission statement every year while you are in school and for the first 5 years after you graduate ... and periodically thereafter, particularly during career transitions. If you are like most people, you'll need to tweak and refine your statement as your talents and passions emerge over time.

Now that you have some clarity about who you are, what you do best, and what makes you happiest, you need a plan (Reference 1). Without a plan, you are leaving the outcome to chance. Yes, your

**Box 1.** Uncover your life's vocation.

Here are some things you should do to uncover your life's vocation:

1. Take an inventory of your talents and skills. Write down the things you believe you are good at—not just subjects at school, but tasks you do at home, with friends, and at work. Think broadly and holistically. Then, narrow down your inventory to more specific tasks under your broad themes. For example, if you're "good with technology," make a list of specific ways you're particularly adept, such as doing Web design, setting up networks, or figuring out how to use complex software. Although you undoubtedly have many skills, try to pick those you think are real standouts. You might not consider these "talents" just yet, but with some time and cultivation, they could be.

2. Take an inventory of your passions. Write down all the things you love to do. Think broadly and holistically. Think about your experiences, and wander through your childhood. Focus on the things you REALLY enjoy(ed), not the things that give you satisfaction because you do them well.

3. Find out what others consider your skills and talents. Ask your family, friends, and colleagues the following questions: What do you think I'm really good at? What are my best qualities or attributes? How would you describe the value or benefit I bring to our family (or our friendship or this organization)? Gather each of their answers in writing.

4. Find the overlaps, and analyze the data. Sit down with your lists. Where do your skills, talents, and passions converge with what others need and perceive about you? Are some themes particularly strong? Are there any surprises? Is there anything missing from what others said about you and what you expected to hear? Are there things you want to explore further with your family, friends, and colleagues? Considering talking it over with someone whose wise counsel you value.

**Box 2.** Writing your personal mission statement.

Writing a personal mission statement will help you discover how you'll use your skills, talents, and passions to make positive contributions to the people closest to you, your community, the profession of pharmacy, and the world. It's not a detailed plan, but rather, a general statement of intent. If calling it a personal mission statement sounds much too serious and somber to you, just call it a personal manifesto, quest, or declaration. To get the process started, here are some things to ponder:

1. Reflect on your vocation. What is your life's journey?
2. What do you value most? If you could invite any three people (living or dead) to your home for dinner, who would you invite and why? What qualities do they possess that inspire you the most?
3. Think about the person you want to become. If you had unlimited time and resources and could be assured you'd be successful, what would you do? What would you like people to say at the lifelong achievement award ceremony held in your honor?
4. How would you like others to perceive you? What type of image would you like to project?

Allow your mind to deeply consider each of these questions, and write down everything that comes to mind. Be open-minded. Don't limit your thinking to what is "doable" or dismiss thoughts that are "unattainable" or "silly."

For further inspiration:

5. Gather some quotes from famous people that really resonate with you.
6. Search the Internet and read the personal mission statements written by other people. There are many great Web sites out there.
7. Ask a trusted adviser to share his or her personal mission statement with you. You can see mine at: www.pharmacy.umaryland.edu/faculty/shaines.

This process might take several days or weeks. Eventually, you'll need to put pencil to paper, or pull out your laptop computer to write. Your mission statement does not need to conform to a particular set of rules. Most statements are succinct declarations—typically, a few sentences. You could express your statement in paragraph form, a bulleted list, a sonnet, or a letter. If creativity isn't your thing, you can always use a template you've discovered on the Internet. Franklin Covey has a "Mission Statement Builder" Web site (available at www.franklincovey.com/msb) that asks you a series of questions and then e-mails you a draft statement that you can then tweak and refine.

personal mission statement will provide guiding principles that can help you set priorities and make better decisions, but a plan of action will help increase the odds for success. Unfortunately, there are lots of overqualified, underemployed pharmacy graduates. But even during tough economic times, some graduates find stellar opportunities and land the postgraduate training program of their choice. The difference between those who are most successful and those who struggle to find employment is not raw talent or dumb luck. It is a carefully considered and well-executed plan. Formulating a plan as early as possible will help you take advantage of opportunities that form the building blocks of your career. Just as a contractor uses an architectural plan, you need to map a path for your professional journey. In addition to developing a plan for how to perform well academically (see Step II – Make the Grade), you should carefully consider how employment, summer internships, extracurricular activities, professional associations, research projects, and elective coursework will help you achieve your personal mission. Your actions for the next few years will send a strong signal to prospective postgraduate training programs and future employers about your commitment. Think about it. If you were a residency or fellowship program director, would you select the candidate whose only evidence of commitment was a passionately expressed, well-worded essay about how a residency would enhance the candidate's career? Or would you pick the person who has shown her commitment by participating in relevant experiences that required initiative, dedication, and resourcefulness? Personally, I'd want the candidate who has a proven record of achievement outside the classroom. Moreover, candidates with diverse experiences bring something of value that they can contribute to the training program and the organization.

So what should your plan look like and what should it include? The fundamental step in creating a plan is developing SMART goals: S = specific, M = measurable, A = attainable, R = relevant, and T = time-bound (Reference 2). Box 3 explains how to write SMART goals. I encourage my students and faculty colleagues to write a list of the SMART goals they want to achieve in the next 6–12 months. Goals should be new commitments, not reiterations of existing obligations. For example, "finish all of the required courses in the spring semester" isn't really a new goal. It was something you were already required to do as part of your degree. The number of new goals you should set depends on their complexity, their difficulty, and your ongoing obligations. From 5 to 10 goals is reasonable. Trying to accomplish more than 10 new goals in 12 months is probably unrealistic. Once you begin to work on a goal, it's a good idea to break it down even more. List the general tactics and

**Box 3**. Writing SMART goals.

Each year, you should develop a list of SMART goals that you will commit to working toward. These goals should be congruent with your personal mission statement and help you achieve your long-term ambitions. A SMART goal should be:

1. **Specific.** Write a declaration of what you plan to accomplish. It should be clear and unambiguous. For example, "contribute to a clinical research project," "gain experience making intravenous (IV) admixtures," "earn an A in the therapeutics course."

2. **Measurable.** How will you know if you have achieved your goal? In some cases, your statement might already include a metric of success. For example, "earn an A in the therapeutics course" contains a specific criterion by which to judge success, namely earning an A. But you may need to embellish your goal statement slightly to include a measurable outcome. For example, "contribute to a clinical research project by assisting with the recruitment and data gathering for 20 subjects."

3. **Attainable.** It's important that your goal be achievable, but not so easily accomplished that it requires minimal effort. Your goal should stretch you and feel challenging. For example, "gain experience making IV admixtures by producing two antibiotic piggybacks and one total parenteral nutrition bag" is probably not challenging enough and doesn't really meet the intent of the underlying aim, namely "gaining experience." Conversely, "conduct a randomized clinical trial examining the impact on diabetes-related outcomes caused by genetic polymorphism related to metformin" isn't achievable, at least not in the next 6–18 months. A trusted adviser can give you feedback on what is an appropriate challenge and what is perhaps unattainable.

4. **Relevant.** Your goal should be relevant to your future aspirations. How does this fit with your overall, long-term plan? Will it help show your commitment to the field? Will it improve your chances of success in your vocation? Some things are probably a better fit than others. For example, if your calling is to become a clinical pharmacy specialist working with patients in ambulatory care settings, "contribute to a clinical research project by running > 50 HPLC samples" probably isn't the best fit. But it might be relevant if you envision that you'll be actively engaged in developing new point-of-care tests to monitor drug therapies. Again, ask a trusted adviser to help you sort out what's most relevant.

> 5. **Time-bound.** Goal statements should make a specific reference to time. When do you plan to accomplish this goal? Planning requires good time management. A goal without a "due date" is less likely to be done. Moreover, thoughtfully reflecting on which goals need to be accomplished first and which can be put off until later in the year will help organize your time and keep you on track. For example, "contribute to a clinical research project by assisting with the recruitment and data gathering for 20 subjects between November 1 and March 1" provides a specific time to accomplish the goal.
>
> HPLC = high-performance liquid chromatography; SMART = specific, measurable, attainable, relevant, and time-bound.

concrete tasks you need to do to achieve the goal. For example, if your goal is to "obtain experience doing clinical research," then "discuss research opportunities with my professors" would be a tactic, and "set up a meeting with Dr. Smith about her patient education study" would be a specific task. Every week, look over your goals, tactics, and tasks. Note what progress (if any) has been made, and ask yourself, what's the next step I need to take to move me forward toward the goal? You don't have to tackle all of your goals simultaneously. Some goals may be prerequisite to other goals. Some goals may naturally be synergistic and best handled at the same time. But, to be successful, you need to make slow yet steady progress. Your weekly reviews will help ensure that you're doing something every week, no matter how small, that's moving you toward your goals.

> *Now that it's all over, what did you really do yesterday that's worth mentioning?*
>
> —Coleman Cox, *Straight Talk from Coleman Cox*

Goals are statements of commitment, not obligation. You will undoubtedly run into roadblocks along the way that either delay your progress or make a goal no longer attainable. No harm lies in tossing a goal that can no longer be accomplished. Every 6–12 months, it's time to take stock of what you've accomplished and to revisit your goals. You may be fortunate enough to have achieved all the goals you've set, but don't be disheartened if a couple of things are left undone. If work is left to do on a goal that you've made good progress toward, it should remain on your list. If your enthusiasm for a particular goal has waned or the goal no longer seems relevant, cross it off. Create new SMART goals. You should develop a habit of creating and revising your professional and personal goals on an annual basis. Many people conduct their annual review at the beginning of the academic year. Others like to do it around the New Year holiday. Set aside a time that seems to work best for you based on your level of enthusiasm and schedule.

## MANAGING YOU

A rigorous pharmacy curriculum will build your knowledge and skills with respect to a breadth of health and medication-related issues. You'll learn the norms of behavior and the ways to be a professional. Developing your knowledge, skill, and attitudes is critically important to your future success as a pharmacist. But, perhaps equally important, cultivating a growth mindset and habits of mind will serve you in all aspects of your life—personal and professional.

A mindset is a set of assumptions held by one or more people that is so well established that it powerfully influences individual and collective behaviors and choices (Reference 3). This pervasive view of the world might be called a "philosophy of life" or "worldview." It is a fundamental cognitive orientation. For example, in the United States, a widely held and fundamental belief is that personal liberty, the freedom of individuals to have control over their own actions without interference from coercion or societal compulsion, is sacrosanct. This belief influences our personal and collective behaviors and our choices in many, many ways. Now, there may be disagreement about what the limits of personal freedom are, the role of government, and the necessity of collective action to advance the common good, but fundamentally, most Americans believe that personal liberty should not be infringed on unless there is darn good reason. This belief has guided us since the founding of our nation.

Carol Dweck, a renowned psychologist at Stanford University, has written extensively about mindset and the ways it influences our motivation and intellectual development (Reference 4). According to Dweck, each of us has a particular mindset with respect to our view about where our talents and successes are derived. On the one extreme, a person with a "fixed mindset" believes success is based on innate ability. Intelligence and talents are fixed traits. We are born with a certain amount, and success will be determined by innate ability. People with a fixed mindset believe they have talents in some areas of their lives, but not in others. That's that. Your intelligence or creativity can't be changed. If you're lucky enough to be born with extraordinary intelligence and creativity, you are destined to do great things. On the other extreme is a "growth mindset," a belief that intelligence and creativity are developed incrementally. Our talents and abilities are not innate, but rather, our success is only limited by steadfast persistence. Most of us fall somewhere in between these two extremes. Sure, not everyone is going to be as successful in business as Warren Buffet, as smart as Steven Hawking, or as fast as Usain Bolt, but we can get wealthier, smarter, or faster *with effort*. Most people are unaware of their mindset, but their cognitive orientation toward intelligence and talent strongly influences behavior, particularly their response to failure. Individuals with a fixed mindset dread failure because it draws attention to and reinforces their beliefs regarding their basic abilities. Therefore, people with a fixed mindset avoid situations in which they might fail. People with a growth mindset do not view failure as an indictment of their fundamental ability. Rather, they are introspective about what they can do to be successful in the future. Failure represents an opportunity for growth. People with a fixed mindset believe that success comes to others without much effort. Failures are signs that their innate ability has been exceeded or has been inadequately rewarded and recognized. A lack of success is not a product of one's own doing, but rather, one's inherent limitations or the failure of others to give us our due. Box 4 gives examples of how people with fixed versus growth mindsets respond differently to failure.

> *My dad encouraged us to fail. Growing up, he would ask us what we failed at that week. If we didn't have something, he would be disappointed. It changed my mindset at an early age that failure is not the outcome. Failure is not trying.*
>
> —Sara Blakely, American businesswoman and youngest self—made female billionaire

Your mindset has profound implications on the likelihood of your achieving your career goals. If talent and intelligence were fixed, then we would see an equal number of successful people in every field with fixed and growth mindsets, based on an assumption that there is about an equal number of each in this world. Why? Because success would be determined by innate abilities, not mindset. But if success were determined by hard work and constructively dealing with failure, then a growth mindset would be the dominant worldview among successful

> **Box 4.** Fixed vs. growth mindset—response to failure.
>
> **Fixed Mindset**
> - "I so deserved an A. I'm smarter than most of the people in this class. That professor is totally arbitrary and asks nitpicky stuff on her exams."
> - "No one will vote for me. I don't like that political stuff anyway."
> - "I think Mary should do the literature search. She's really good at it, and I want to do well on this project."
> - "Maybe you should conduct the patient interview. I really flubbed it up last time."
>
> **Growth Mindset**
> - "I'm really upset I got a B. I probably should have read that article on the recommended reading list."
> - "I really hope I win the election, but if I don't, I know my chances are better next time."
> - "Do you mind if I do the initial literature search on this project? It's something I need to work on. Mary, I'd really like your feedback. You did a great job on our last project."
> - "I'm sorry I screwed up last time. I think I'm better prepared for the patient interview today."

people. Indeed, Dr. Dweck has shown precisely that; a person with a growth mindset is more likely to achieve success. And those who are successful are more likely to possess a growth mindset.

What do people with a growth mindset do to help them achieve success? They embrace challenges, persist in the face of obstacles, seek and learn from criticism, and view effort as necessary for improvement. Moreover, those with a growth mindset are inspired by the success of others and often seek the advice of role models and mentors. Can we move our mindset toward growth? Ironically, those with a truly fixed mindset may be unable to do so. Luckily, most of us are not that extreme, and there are ways to build your growth mindset. First, become aware of your mindset. You can take a mindset survey (available at http://mindsetonline.com/testyourmindset/step1.php) to determine your general tendencies. When you face challenging decisions, be mindful of your tendencies, and purposely take the steps that will foster growth. Of course, it all sounds very simple, but in reality, it can be quite scary to do something beyond what you perceive is your capacity or where the chance of failure seems too high. Again, mentors and friends who have a growth mindset can give you the emotional support to take on new challenges you feel are beyond your reach. Conversely, you don't want to take foolhardy risks. But your trusted advisers should be able to steer you away from danger.

In addition to adopting a growth mindset, it's important to develop habits of mind that will increase your chances of success. Steven Covey's popular book titled *The 7 Habits of Highly Effective People: Powerful Lessons in Personal Change* is perhaps one of the most influential self-help books regarding how to lead a productive and balanced life (Reference 5). I encourage you to read it. In a similar vein, Arthur Costa described 12 essential characteristics for success, which were subsequently expanded (Reference 6) (see Box 5). These habits are ways of thinking that people employ to solve complex and challenging problems. These habits of mind build on the concept of mindset, and they describe how successful people respond when the answer or the "right" choice is not readily apparent. Although each of these habits may seem intuitively good, they are not skills that most of us naturally possess; they must be cultivated and nurtured. If we are fortunate, our parents, elementary and high school teachers, and undergraduate professors instilled these habits of mind. How do we develop them further? Mindful practice! Developing an awareness of what these habits are and deploying them in our daily lives. You may already possess strong habits

---

**Box 5.** Habits of mind.

- Managing impulsivity
- Listening with understanding and empathy
- Thinking flexibly
- Thinking about thinking
- Striving for accuracy
- Questioning and posing problems
- Applying past knowledge to new situations
- Thinking and communicating with clarity and precision
- Gathering data through all senses
- Creating, imagining, innovating
- Responding with wonderment and awe
- Taking responsible risks
- Finding humor
- Thinking interdependently
- Remaining open to continuous learning

in some areas. For example, you might be really good about listening to others with understanding and empathy, thinking and communicating with clarity and precision, striving for accuracy and precision, and applying past knowledge to new situations. But you may not be so good at managing impulsivity (e.g., jumping to conclusions without gathering all the facts), gathering data through all senses (e.g., poor observational skills), or thinking flexibly (e.g., failing to consider alternative viewpoints). Another skill that many of us fail to fully develop is thinking about our thinking; reflecting on and evaluating the quality of our own thoughts and mental strategies. Few think about their learning strategies when confronted with a particularly difficult subject or reflect back on an experience, particularly when the outcome was positive. To cultivate your habits of mind, place yourself in circumstances that require you to mindfully engage these habits. Group work will help you develop your habits in the areas of thinking interdependently while listening to others and thinking flexibly. Writing a scientific paper would probably help you develop your ability to communicate with clarity, strive for accuracy, and learn continuously. As you strengthen your growth mindset, you will naturally want to engage in activities that foster these habits of mind. In turn, these habits will help you accomplish your goals and achieve success.

## PLANNING YOUR CAREER

> *I cannot stress too much the need for self-invention. To be authentic is literally to be your own author ... to discover your own native energies and desires, and then to find your own way of acting on them.*
>
> —Warren Bennis, *On Becoming a Leader*

One of the challenges you will face throughout your career is making good decisions, ones that will lead you closer to your goals and express your vocation. At this stage in your development, you may be wondering what type of postgraduate training program is right for you. Not only will you need to decide which training path is best, but you will also need to decide which program(s) (see Table 1). A growing number of pharmacy graduates are pursuing residency training, and it is increasingly an expected credential by employers and professional associations (Reference 7). Residency training programs are intended to increase your confidence and skill as a practitioner (Reference 8). Postgraduate year one (PGY1) programs are conducted in almost all patient care settings, including community pharmacies, community-based clinics, hospitals, long-term care facilities, and managed care organizations. During a PGY1 residency, the focus is on foundational skills, including direct patient care activities, information mastery, practice management, and project management. A postgraduate year two (PGY2) residency is intended to build on these skills, with a focus on a specific patient population or pharmacy practice management. PGY1 programs may employ only a single resident and a few preceptors or may be large programs with more than a dozen residents and many preceptors. A PGY2 residency training program typically has only one or two residency positions and relatively few specialists who serve as the core set of preceptors. The advantage of a small program is that you often receive individualized attention. The disadvantages may include a lack of opportunity to interact with other residents, preceptors with a narrower range of expertise, and limited elective options. Residency training programs with a long record of excellence often receive hundreds of applications each year, and it can be difficult to land an interview or match with these programs. Don't let the potential odds dissuade you from applying for a program that matches with your vocational aspirations and for which you are well prepared. With a growth mindset, you know that success comes from preparation and learning from setbacks.

The types of experiences that will prepare you to be a well-qualified residency candidate are discussed in detail throughout this field guide: academic performance; organizational involvement; patient care and practice-related experiences through work and school; scholarship and research; and networking. Developing a thoughtful plan and documenting your professional development activities will position you for success.

Residency program directors and preceptors expect residents to enter their programs with a strong knowledge base regarding the therapeutic use of medications as well as previous experience interviewing patients, documenting patient encounters, and participating on patient care teams. If you have the opportunity to take elective didactic courses in areas of advanced therapeutics like cardiology, critical care, infectious diseases, oncology, pediatrics, or women's health (to name a few), these courses will not only enhance your knowledge regarding the therapeutics of drugs but will also show your commitment to patient care as a foundational element of your vocation. Moreover, it is important to seek rigorous introductory and advanced practice experiences that give you many opportunities to interact directly with patients such as conducting interviews, performing physical examinations, and documenting your findings. Participating in team-based care activities in multiple environments is also a big plus.

**Table 1.** Postgraduate Training Options

| | Residency | Fellowship | Graduate Degree |
|---|---|---|---|
| **Key features** | Mix of practice-based experiences to build the skills and confidence needed to manage patients and a practice | Mix of research experiences conducting basic, translational, or clinical research | Curriculum of didactic courses and experiences; the intended outcome is program-specific |
| **Setting** | Any practice setting | Academic health sciences center, college or university, pharmaceutical industry[a] | College or university |
| **Typical duration (years)** | 1–2 | 1[b]–3 | 2–5 |
| **Key benefits** | • Enhance your patient care and practice management skills.<br>• Growing expectation by employers that entry-level pharmacists have completed a residency | • Learn research design and statistics.<br>• Develop grant writing skills.<br>• Build a research portfolio. | • Deep acquisition of knowledge and skill<br>• Degree awarded |
| **Potential drawbacks** | • Some preceptors may not be experienced teachers or mentors.<br>• Program may not be affiliated with an academic institution. | • Often, a single mentor and a few preceptors | • Tuition<br>• Salary often depends on obtaining a teaching or research assistantship. |

| | | | |
|---|---|---|---|
| **Key factors to consider** | • Type of practice model and the patient population(s) served<br>• Duration (years in existence) and size (number of residents) of the program<br>• Quality and depth of services and preceptors<br>• Opportunities for teaching and formal teaching certificate program?<br>• Accredited?[c] | • Type of research methods and experiences<br>• Scholarly record of program director<br>• Resources and funding for independent research project<br>• Opportunities for teaching?<br>• Peer reviewed or other quality credential? | • Scholarly record and interests of program faculty |
| **Preparing yourself** | • Take elective courses that align with your vocational vision.<br>• Obtain strong direct patient care experiences in a variety of settings and populations.<br>• Gain leadership experience, both formal and informal.<br>• Have a record of employment doing pharmacy or health-related work. | • Take elective courses that align with your vocational vision.<br>• Obtain research experiences in a variety of settings.<br>• Participate as an author on a scholarly paper.<br>• Consider completing a PGY1 residency first. | • Take elective courses that align with your vocational vision.<br>• Consider concurrently completing a residency. |

[a] Some industry-based "fellowship" programs do not focus on developing research skills; these programs might best be described as postgraduate internships.
[b] The American College of Clinical Pharmacy recommends that fellowship programs be a minimum of 2 years so that the fellow can fully develop the necessary research skills and complete a scholarly project.
[c] Completing an unaccredited residency training program will affect your PGY2 residency training options and board certification through the Board of Pharmacy Specialties.

PGY1 = postgraduate year one; PGY2 = postgraduate year two.

Gaining leadership experience will prepare you for residency training and for life (Reference 9). Now, you might be thinking that leadership is all about becoming an elected officer in a student organization. Certainly, this is one manifestation. But leadership occurs when one person exerts influence and enlists the support of others to accomplish a common goal. Yes, there are leaders with formal titles who have been vested with certain authority to marshal the collective actions of a group. Examples include organizational presidents, committee chairs, project managers, and lead technicians. Each has been tasked with accomplishing specific, often predetermined goals. But not everyone with a formal title is a leader. Indeed, we've all witnessed examples in which the formal leader's style and decisions have not only failed to create a path toward a desired goal that others might walk, but have also left a pile of debris on a trail of destruction.

Leadership is not about title; rather, it is about positively influencing the actions of groups. Indeed, you can lead without being in charge. All of us have the power to influence others. You exert power when we encourage and assist others who share your vision. You exert power when you possess technical knowledge and expertise that others value and need. You exert power through the force of your character by building goodwill, trustworthiness, and respect.

The opportunities are unlimited for you to develop your leadership skills. Leadership opportunities exist at school, work, and home and within professional societies, fraternities, religious organizations, and civic groups. One of the obvious prerequisites of leadership is to be a member of a group. Thus, belonging to and being an active participant in the work of a group is a minimal first step toward leadership. Perhaps one of the easiest ways to build your leadership skills is to volunteer to organize a group project at school or work. Read about leadership strategies and use them to forge a common commitment with your group. Reflect on each leadership experience and think about what worked well and what didn't. Everyone has his or her own leadership style, a preferred approach to working with groups (see Table 2). Discover your leadership style and cultivate it. After you've volunteered to lead groups in informal ways and gained experience, formal leadership opportunities will quickly come your way. People will begin to recognize your skills and seek you out. Indeed, you may get overwhelmed by the many leadership opportunities presented to you. It's important to be selective; pick the opportunities that best align with your passions and vocational aspirations. (For more information, see Step IV – Develop Leadership and Management Abilities.)

**Table 2.** Leadership Styles

| Style | Description |
|---|---|
| Authoritarian | Keeps close control over followers by establishing strict rules, procedures, and organizational structures. Supervises followers closely |
| Coaching | Encourages self-development and empowers followers to act independently. Tries to link the personal goals of followers with the organizational goals |
| Democratic | Encourages shared decision-making through discussion and debate. Believes in social equality and that everyone should play a role in the group's decisions |
| Laissez-faire | Establishes goals but delegates responsibilities and tasks to followers, allowing them a high degree of autonomy. Provides materials necessary to accomplish the goal but does not directly participate in decision-making |
| Transactional | Motivates followers through a system of rewards and, occasionally, punishments. Seeks to maintain order by working within the organizational culture |
| Transformative | Seeks to change the status quo. Inspires others by articulating a clear vision and role modeling desired behaviors. Encourages followers to put group interests first |

Finally, a strong track record of employment will enhance your chances of landing a great postgraduate training position. A record of employment doing incrementally more challenging work is an indicator that you will be valuable employee. Moreover, it suggests that you have good time management skills and are able to prioritize your responsibilities in a manner that allows you to be successful at school and work. Employment in pharmacy or health-related institutions is often symbiotic with your academic studies. What you see, do, and learn through your employment will help you see the relevance of what is being taught in the classroom. And vice versa; what you learn in class can be applied at your work. Employment provides additional opportunity to practice leadership and gain experience with direct patient care. (For more information, see Step V – Gain Valuable Work Experience.)

In summary, your academic record, organizational involvement, patient care experiences, employment history, engagement in scholarly projects, and professional network are all ways to set yourself apart from other residency and fellowship candidates. Developing and implementing a plan will help you set priorities and maximize your potential (see Table 3). Your commitment is expressed through these endeavors, and these activities can be synergistic when they align with your vocational goals. Moreover, these activities will help you build relationships that will become your professional network. The most important and powerful letters of recommendation you garner will most likely be written by professors, organizational leaders, and work supervisors who've witnessed your talents and can attest to your commitment.

## FINDING A MENTOR

Mentoring is a symbiotic relationship in which a knowledgeable and respected person in a profession or organization nurtures and assists a less experienced person who shares common interests (Reference 10). Research has found a strong correlation between the presence of a mentoring relationship and career satisfaction and success. Mentoring relationships are of mutual benefit; each seeks to advance the career objectives of the other. The mentor encourages the mentee by recognizing strengths, acknowledging successes, and inviting participation in activities that align with their mutual career goals. A mentor teaches by providing feedback and helping the mentee acquire the knowledge, skill, and attitudes needed to succeed. In addition, mentors use their professional standing to sponsor the junior person by making introductions to influential members of the profession, creating employment opportunities, and vouching for the mentee's great ability. A mentor counsels by actively listening, asking probing questions, and providing sound advice. Thus, there are many potential benefits to developing a mentoring relationship with one of your professors, supervisors, or role models.

    In a healthy mentoring relationship, the person being mentored is not a parasite living off the "good graces" of the mentor. Rather, the mentee contributes to the mentor's work in meaningful ways. The mentee, for example, might provide technical assistance to the mentor with patient care, teaching, research, or service activities. Indeed, mentoring relationships most often arise from a task related to the mentor's work responsibilities. During the initial weeks of the relationship, the mentor and mentee begin to identify their mutual interests and extend welcoming messages to one another. The mentee expresses a strong desire to be coached, and the mentor invites more interaction. During the cultivation stage of the relationship, there is frequent and meaningful collaboration. The mentor often gains a revitalized sense of self-esteem and a renewed interest in work. Although the relationship revolves around professional goals and tasks, a personal dimension often emerges. The mentor and mentee develop an emotional bond; each cares deeply about the other's personal and professional success. I've had the good fortune to have great mentors in my life and the opportunity to mentor others. Like a friendship, cultivating a mentoring relationship starts with mutual interests and an invitation. Many schools assign students to academic advisers, often with little regard to the professional interests of the student—or the professor, for that matter. Although these preassigned advising relationships occasionally work out, most do not. But nothing prevents you from proactively seeking someone else. There may even be mechanisms at your school to officially switch your academic advisor. There is nothing more flattering to a professor or senior practitioner than to have someone less experienced seek his or her advice and wisdom. Through your coursework, employment, or leadership activities, you will encounter people you admire whose work seems to align with your interests. Set up an appointment to talk about their career path. If the encounter flows well and you leave with a good vibe, seek other opportunities to interact by suggesting that you participate in a meaningful task together. It's that simple. You can't force someone to be your mentor, but you can create the conditions for a mentoring relationship to develop.

> As a pharmacy student I wish I had developed relationships with more of the faculty. It wasn't until my fourth year that I realized the importance of great mentors.
>
> —Lauren Biehle, 2011/12 PGY2 Pharmacy Resident at University of Houston College of Pharmacy/Cardinal Health, Houston, Tex.

The typical mentor is 10–20 years older than the mentee. Most mentor-mentee pairs are the same sex. This doesn't mean that mentoring relationships between people who are only 5 years apart in professional seniority and the opposite sex don't exist, but there are potential pitfalls to consider. One potential problem pertains to the emotional dimensions of the relationship; a love interest might emerge. All too often, these quasi-mentoring relationships end on a very sour note, negatively affecting both individuals personally and professionally. Mid-career mentors who are in their "professional prime" are better able to serve as mentors because they often have a large network and greater knowledge of profession-wide trends. Late-career mentors often have an elevated standing within the profession and may be motivated by a strong desire to leave a legacy. Developing a mentoring relationship

**Table 3.** Recommended Career-Building Activities by Professional Year

| Professional Year | Recommended Career-Building Activity |
| --- | --- |
| P1 | • Join a professional pharmacy organization like the American Pharmacists Association – Academy of Student Pharmacists.<br>• Seek part-time employment as a pharmacy technician.<br>• Talk to faculty and pharmacy leaders about their career path.<br>• Write a personal mission statement.<br>• Develop five SMART goals.<br>• Lead one school-, work-, or professional organization–related project.<br>• Consider a summer internship with the pharmaceutical industry, the U.S. Public Health Service, or a research organization. |
| P2 | • Revisit and refine your personal mission statement.<br>• Review your progress toward your goals; develop 5–10 new SMART goals.<br>• Join a specialty organization (e.g., ACCP, American Society of Consultant Pharmacists, Society of Critical Care Medicine, American Diabetes Association) that aligns with your vocational goals.<br>• Seek one formal leadership role (elected or appointed) in a student professional organization.<br>• Seek a faculty mentor with whom you share professional interests.<br>• Take elective coursework that matches your vocational goals.<br>• Attend a state pharmacy association meeting, and consider attending a national pharmacy association meeting.<br>• Consider a summer internship, or work full-time as a senior pharmacy technician with expanded responsibilities. |

| | |
|---|---|
| P3 | - Revisit and refine your personal mission statement.
- Review your progress toward your goals; develop 5–10 new SMART goals.
- Meet with your mentor regularly.
- Take elective coursework that matches your vocational goals.
- Participate in a scholarly project.
- Seek a leadership role (elected or appointed) in your school's formal structures, a university-wide organization, or a state pharmacy association.
- Attend a national pharmacy association meeting.
- Seek expanded work responsibilities, including projects related to patient care. |
| P4 | - Revisit and refine your personal mission statement.
- Review your progress toward your goals; develop 5–10 new SMART goals.
- Meet with your mentor regularly.
- Attend a national specialty professional association meeting (one that matches your vocational aspirations).
- Seek advanced practice rotations with a reputation for being rigorous; seek opportunities to interact with patients; and work with interprofessional teams.
- Take advanced practice electives that match your vocational goals. |

ACCP = American College of Clinical Pharmacy; SMART = specific, measurable, attainable, relevant, and time-bound.

with someone who is the same sex makes frank discussions about family relationships and gender roles possible. Mentoring relationships grow organically, and it's difficult to predict whether a strong rapport will develop. Don't be too disappointed if the mentor relationship you're trying to cultivate doesn't seem to flourish the way you'd envisioned. Your potential mentor might not have a nurturing personality or be able to commit enough time to the relationship. Regardless, you will have benefited from your interactions, no matter how brief, with this role model.

> *The greatest good you can do for another is not just to share your riches, but to reveal to him his own.*
> —Benjamin Disraeli, British Prime Minister (1868, 1874—1880)

To be mentored is to be open to the wise counsel of someone more experienced. It does not require you to unquestionably act on every piece of advice you receive, but it does require you to consider it and think flexibly, allowing your mind to change in response to new information. A good mentor will not only congratulate you on your successes but will also point out how your performance can be better. Moreover, a mentor will encourage you to take on challenges you might not feel quite ready for and steer you away from things that might be too risky. A mentor can help you sort out a true growth opportunity that aligns with your vocation goals from what might be a potential waste of your time and talent. By sharing your authentic self with a mentor, you can chart a course together that will increase your chances of professional success and personal satisfaction.

## IT'S A JOURNEY

Becoming a well-qualified residency or fellowship candidate is a journey. Your journey should start by engaging in some introspection, identifying your professional vocation, and selecting a destination. Having a road map will help you get there more efficiently, but remain flexible. There will be roadblocks on your journey. With a growth mindset, you'll turn these obstacles into opportunities. Occasional adventures off the path can lead to the most delightful discoveries, so don't be afraid to change your route. Mentors make good travel companions. They can help interpret the maps, point out the shortcuts, warn you about speed bumps, and show you the sights. Remember to keep a travelog of what you've seen and experienced. And when you arrive at your destination, it will be time to start planning your next trip.

## REFERENCES

1. Johnson V. Goal Setting. 13 Secrets of World Class Achievers. Melrose, FL: No Dream Too Big Publishing, 2012.
2. Gudger J. SMART Goals. The Ultimate Goal Setting Guide. Amazon Digital Services, 2012.
3. Dweck CS. Mindset: The New Psychology of Success. New York: Ballantine Books, 2006.
4. Dweck C. Self-Theories. Available at www.learning-knowledge.com/self-theories.html. Accessed August 29, 2012.
5. Covey SR. The 7 Habits of Highly Effective People: Powerful Lessons in Personal Change. New York: Free Press, 1989.
6. Costa AL, Kallick B, eds. Learning and Leading with Habits of Mind. 16 Essential Characteristics for Success. Alexandria, VA: American Society of Curriculum Development, 2008.
7. Murphy JE, Nappi JM, Bosso JJ, et al. American College of Clinical Pharmacy's vision of the future: postgraduate pharmacy residency training as a prerequisite for direct patient care practice. Pharmacotherapy 2006;26:722–33.
8. Haines ST. Making residency training an expectation for pharmacists in direct patient care roles. Am J Pharm Educ 2007;71:Article 71.
9. Bennis W. On Becoming a Leader. New York: Basic Books, 2003.
10. Haines ST. The mentor-protégé relationship. Am J Pharm Educ 2003;67:Article 82.

# STEP II
# MAKING THE GRADE

Dana P. Hammer, R.Ph., M.S., Ph.D.

## ABBREVIATIONS IN THIS CHAPTER

| | |
|---|---|
| APPE | Advanced pharmacy practice experience |
| CPD | Continuing professional development |
| CPE | Continuing pharmacy education |
| CV | Curriculum vitae |
| IPPE | Introductory pharmacy practice experience |
| RPD | Residency program director |

> CHARLIE BROWN: "Lucy. I am so confused. I have no idea what it is I'm supposed to learn or when I know what I've learned whatever it is I'm supposed to learn. Grades have just come out and I'm afraid to open the envelope with my transcript. How will I know when I've succeeded? How will I know when I've "got it"?
> 
> LUCY: "That's the mystery of education Charlie Brown!"
> 
> CHARLIE BROWN: "Good Grief!"
> 
> —Charles Schulz

## WHY YOU SHOULD READ THIS CHAPTER

Good grief, indeed! The process of learning, and grades denoted to communicate something about that learning, can be very mysterious. As a former residency director, I have read many a transcript and interviewed many a candidate. What are we looking for? Lots of things—the vast majority of which are discussed in this book. With respect to transcripts, many of us look for the various courses that applicants have completed, their grades in these courses as well as their grades in introductory pharmacy practice experiences (IPPEs) and advanced pharmacy practice experiences (APPEs), and their overall GPA. This review can be an important component in our decision to invite applicants to interview.

The title of this chapter may lead you to believe that grades are the focus of pharmacy school. But is the strenuous journey of 3–4 years of professional, doctoral-level education really about achieving grades? Is it only about preparing for a residency? Of course not! "Making the Grade" refers not to a letter or number but to a high level of performance. I can almost guarantee that each of you, in your application and/or admissions interview for pharmacy school, said something to the effect that part of why you want to be a pharmacist is to help people. Helping others implies much, but the core of helping others is sharing and using your knowledge and skills to others' benefit. As such, you need to learn as much as you can and continue that learning beyond graduation to really fulfill this potential. Grades should be simply a notation involved in the learning process. Unfortunately—though understandably—for some students, the achievement of good grades can become their sole focus in pharmacy school. We don't want to minimize the impact that grades can have on your future success: scholarships, admission to residencies, and employment opportunities are all linked to the grades you receive. But you should be most successful if you don't make grades your primary goal. Focus on learning to fulfill your potential as a professional, and your grades should reflect your effort.

> *As a pharmacy student, I wish I had lost the "I'll never use this" attitude when learning about certain things in the classroom. Whether it's learning about different diagnostic tests, a specific specialty area, or even some of those biochemistry reactions that you swear you'll never see again, they usually creep up and surprise you at least once during residency.*
>
> —Alexander H. Flannery, 2011/12 PGY1 Pharmacy Practice Resident at Medical University of South Carolina, Charleston, S.C.

## BECOMING A SELF-DIRECTED LEARNER AND STUDYING FOR UNDERSTANDING

You may have heard that information and knowledge are increasing so rapidly that much of what you learn now will be obsolete in, say, less than 5 years. If this is true, then it is imperative that we focus more on how we learn, and less on what we learn, so that we can keep up with the knowledge and information affecting our profession. Self-directed learning has been defined as follows:

a process in which individuals take the initiative, with or without the help of others, in diagnosing learning needs, formulating goals, identifying human and material resources for learning, choosing and implementing appropriate learning strategies, and evaluating learning outcomes. (Reference 1)

Many pharmacy school curricula are helping students develop these skills through techniques such as problem-based or team-based learning. In these models, students must determine what information they need to find and synthesize to answer certain questions or solve specific problems. This model is quite different from that of passively listening to lectures, per se, in which the knowledge you need is given to you. Both educational techniques have merit in pharmacy school curricula. The former, however, is more likely to develop skills that will carry you into your future practice: how to determine what you need to know and then how to find and apply that information.

Even if much of your pharmacy school curriculum is passive and lecture-based, here are some tips to help you become a self-directed learner in the pharmacy academic setting:

- **Ask yourself how the information affects your ability to care for patients and practice pharmacy, either directly or indirectly.** If you don't know, then try to find out. Write down the connections you discover. We know from education research that writing and applying the content improves our ability to retain information.
- **Study with others.** Many students discover value in sharing notes as well as conversing with and quizzing others about the material because you may have different learning styles and ways of interpreting information. Create learning communities around your different courses.
- **Study for understanding.** In a lecture and examination-based course, it is easy to engage in what some call the "binge-and-purge" method of learning—cram knowledge into your head for quick recall on an exam. This technique may help you survive yet another exam, but it does not necessarily help you understand and apply the material. Not to mention that this method of "learning" may make subsequent courses more difficult since the prerequisite knowledge you were supposed to gain was not retained. Asking yourself the first question in this list, creating meaning about the information and determining how it could be used, will help you gain a much better and lingering understanding of the material. This understanding should help you become a better practitioner,

since your knowledge has been stored in an "applied" context—you don't just know a bunch of facts, you know how to use that information to help patients.
- **Talk with your instructors and preceptors.** Ask them to suggest ways in which you can better learn and understand their material (or be better prepared for your responsibilities, in the case of experiential learning with preceptors) and meet their objectives. You can also ask them any other questions you have while you're at it! Faculty and preceptors appreciate engaged, inquisitive students. This interaction can also go a long way in helping you build mentoring relationships with them. Your instructors and preceptors are there to help you become a competent, professional practitioner. Take advantage of their expertise and wisdom while you can.

In the end, becoming a self-directed learner is really about motivating yourself to learn as much as you can. It's easy to become complacent about learning, especially when curricula are heavy and intense and you don't have much free time outside the class/rotation, your work, your family responsibilities, and the like. Continually striving to learn, however, should help you perform better not only in pharmacy school, but also during your residency and in your future practice.

## CONTINUING PROFESSIONAL DEVELOPMENT AND CONTINUING PHARMACY EDUCATION: THE IMPORTANCE OF LIFELONG LEARNING

As you have likely been told, pharmacists must continually seek learning opportunities to keep up with changes in practice and be fully prepared to serve patients and other health care providers. This is another hallmark of being a professional. Continuing professional development (CPD) is essentially self-directed learning after graduation that includes continuing pharmacy education (CPE). CPE is a model of post-graduation learning whereby pharmacists must obtain a certain number of "hours" or credits of continuing education courses to maintain currency of their licenses to practice pharmacy. These hours are often obtained via live continuing education courses offered at pharmacy conferences, as well as via courses offered through the Internet. The CPE model is not unlike licensing procedures for many other health professions. There is debate, however, about the effectiveness of such a system to keep practitioners current in their knowledge and motivated in their learning.

Continuing pharmacy education is considered a component of CPD. The CPD cycle (Figure 1) is similar to self-directed learning because it prompts pharmacists to:

> reflect on their practice and assess their knowledge and skills, identify learning needs, create a personal learning plan, implement the learning plan, and evaluate the effectiveness of the educational interventions and the plan in relation to their practice. (Reference 2)

Continuing pharmacy education could be the educational interventions in the CPD cycle. Authors suggest that the CPD cycle should be continuous versus episodic to have the most impact on a pharmacist's practice. Traditional CPE could be episodic for some pharmacists—for instance, if all required credit hours are obtained in one weekend conference. My use of the CPD cycle looks like this:

- **Reflect** – what questions have I been asked in the pharmacy that I struggled to answer without looking up further information? What sorts of CPE programs have I *not* participated in in awhile? What topics would I like to learn more about to better serve my practice or pursue new avenues in practice? I also set learning goals for myself for these topics.
- **Plan** – at what conferences can I find the topics I identified in my reflection? Are there online or journal based programs on these topics if I am unable to find appropriate conferences? How do I build those into my schedule?
- **Act** – participate in the conference, or online or journal based programs, preferably throughout the year. Document participation and learning in a portfolio (or at this time, a file of CPE programs in which I participated).
- **Evaluate** – for me, this is really part of the reflection process. Did my plan for CPE meet my learning objectives? Am I feeling more comfortable in practice with the topics of which I learned more about? Am I pursuing new avenues in my practice based on new knowledge and skills (if that was one of my learning goals)? This reflection/evaluation of my learning helps me to plan for the next set of learning outcomes I want to achieve to continually develop my professional life.

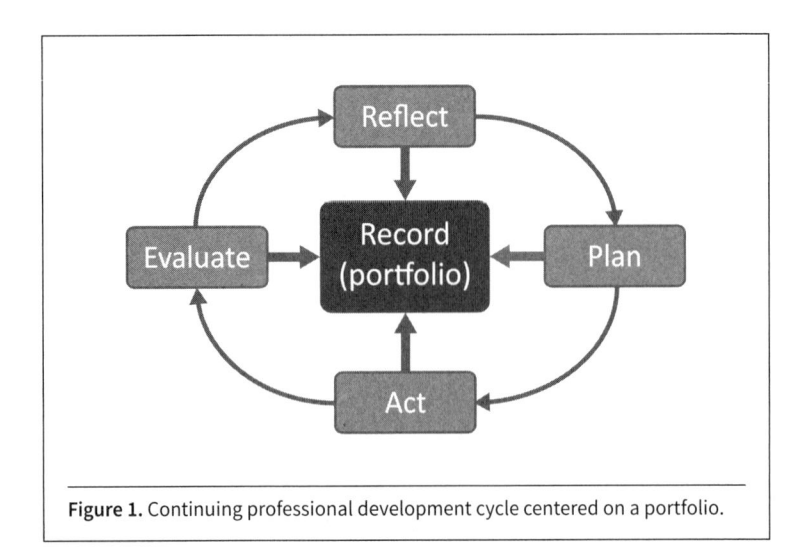

Figure 1. Continuing professional development cycle centered on a portfolio.

The Accreditation Council for Pharmacy Education offers a set of tools to assist practitioners with each phase of the cycle (Reference 3). At least one pharmacy school has implemented the cycle in the first year of its curriculum (Reference 4).

Regardless of how continuing education is obtained, the important point is that all professionals should become lifelong learners. Becoming a self-directed learner during pharmacy school should continue throughout your career. Learning does not end with graduation. On the contrary, it is critical that we keep up with current knowledge and skills to best serve our patients and colleagues in practice. The desire to learn to improve your knowledge for the betterment of your practice is paramount in providing the best care for your patients.

## THE RELATIONSHIP OF GRADES TO LEARNING

You have likely lived with grades your entire academic career—in fact, it is very likely that your good grades helped you get into pharmacy school in the first place! Have you ever taken the time to think about what those grades really mean? What do they say about you and your learning? Many faculty feel that grades provide information about how well students are learning (Reference 5). Walvoord and Anderson discuss grading as a complex process used for:

- **Evaluation:** the grade purports to be a valid, fair, and trustworthy judgment about the quality of the student's work.

- **Communication:** the grade is a communication to the student, as well as to employers, graduate schools, and others. Grading is also the occasion of (sometimes highly emotional) communication and is thus an important and powerful aspect of the ongoing classroom conversation among students and teachers.
- **Motivation:** grading affects how students study, what they focus on, how much time they spend, and how involved they become in the course. Thus grading is a powerful part of the motivational structure of the course, for better or worse.
- **Organization:** a grade on a test or assignment helps mark transitions, bring closure, and focus effort for both students and teachers (Reference 6).

Many factors can contribute to the process of assigning grades. There is also a certain measure of subjectivity in the grades we have been assigned, given that our different teachers and preceptors may have used quite varied criteria for assigning grades. Some people feel that grades may even impede the learning process because the achievement of the grade may seem to become the learner's goal, versus learning to become a more competent professional. Thus, grades do not necessarily provide an entirely accurate and complete picture of our learning. They are merely a judgment at a given point in time.

In addition to the previous discussion regarding grade assignment, some people may view grades as a glimpse into your personality; for some, grades may represent characteristics such as motivation, work ethic, responsibility, goal-orientation, discipline, and the ability to respect authority and seek assistance. Others may consider grades completely arbitrary because of the extreme difficulty in determining exactly what a grade represents. These people may not consider grades at all when making judgments about people. Indeed, grades and the process of grading are quite complex in what they represent.

## SO WHY ARE GRADES IMPORTANT?

Although we know that grades may not be a completely accurate portrayal of your learning, your personality, your potential to succeed, and many other factors, they are still used for making big decisions such as admissions to professional and graduate programs and honor societies—or awarding of financial aid, scholarships, and other awards. Is there evidence that grades affect future practice or help achieve a residency? What if your pharmacy school doesn't award grades? These questions will be discussed in this section, together with the real reasons that studying for understanding (which may translate to high grades!) is critical.

## Do Grades Predict Success in Practice or Residency?

Neither question has been studied much in the pharmacy academy, likely because it is very difficult to do so in a valid and reliable manner. Some studies have assessed the impact of GPA on clerkship performance. Kidd and Latif found that pre-pharmacy GPAs were not predictive of clerkship GPAs, although they did not analyze pharmacy school GPAs against clerkship GPAs in their study (Reference 7). Conversely, Allen and Bond found that pre-pharmacy GPAs were predictive of a combined variable of pharmacy practice and required clerkship course grades (Reference 8). In the general higher education literature, it has been noted:

> The GPA is also a relatively poor basis on which to predict future performance, which perhaps explains why such attempts are never very impressive. In fact, a number of meta-analyses of this relationship, conducted every ten years or so since 1965, reveals that the median correlation between GPA and future performance is 0.18; a value that is neither very useful nor impressive. The strongest relationship between GPA and future achievement is usually found between undergraduate GPA and first-year performance in graduate or professional school. (Reference 9)

Of interest, in the absence of solid evidence about the ability of grades to predict performance in practice, many authors in the pharmacy academy as well as the practice arena have discussed why grades and test scores should not be the only factors in admitting students to pharmacy schools—or in admitting pharmacy students to residency programs. From these discussions, it seems that a well-rounded student would be better prepared for a residency and patient care service than a person who is not.

## Are Grades Important in the Resident Selection Process?

Of the published information that I found, two studies noted that grades are one of the most common criteria by which residency programs select applicants to be invited to interview (References 10, 11). McCollum and Hansen found that in their institution, students who received residencies had higher GPAs than those who did not, although this finding was not statistically significant (Reference 12). Caballero and colleagues noted that "poor academic performance relative to peer applicants" plays a role in "students' inability to secure a residency position," although they also mentioned that some students at their institution who had not obtained residencies had received high grades (Reference 13). Residency faculty from one institution discussed their ranking system in the process of selecting applicants for interviews, which included a review of grades. Presenters noted, however, that several of the institution's residents who had originally scored high in the applicant ranking process did not necessarily perform well during their residency, and vice versa (Reference 14). In the context of using grades as a criterion for selection to a residency program, Jungnickel writes that:

> a number of factors limit the direct comparison of GPAs obtained from different pharmacy schools. Pharmacy schools may differ greatly in program outcomes, both those that are anticipated as well as those that are actually achieved by graduates. Doctor of pharmacy programs also vary greatly in structure and content, including factors such as pre-pharmacy requirements, material taught, teaching and learning approaches, and duration and structure of practice experiences. In addition, grades may have far different meanings at different pharmacy schools. For example, based on curricular and programmatic differences, a 3.5 cumulative GPA at two different pharmacy schools may represent very distinct differences in knowledge and skills. Given the aforementioned factors, a lower-ranked applicant from one school may be better prepared for a particular residency program than a higher-ranked applicant from another school. (Reference 15)

Although robust evidence is lacking about the use of grades in the residency selection process, anecdotal evidence suggests that grades are being used more often by residency programs as "tie breakers" in the initial screening of applications. This practice seems to have grown as a method to evaluate an increasing number of applications. Several residency program directors (RPDs) I queried noted that although grades are not usually heavily weighted in the application screening process, they have become more important in determining who may be selected for an interview, given that competition has increased.

### *What If Your Pharm.D. Program Doesn't Award Grades?*

Some pharmacy schools don't award grades. Their learners are measured on a pass/no-pass basis, having demonstrated a certain level of competence to "pass." Some of these schools may maintain an internal ranking system of how their students compare with each other on the basis of academic achievement. This information may only be available by request, however. So how do RPDs consider these nongraded transcripts in their decision-making process? Although I found no published literature to help answer this question, I learned that some preliminary research shows that even though many residency programs do not necessarily put a lot of weight on applicants' grades in their interview selection process, it is difficult to compare nongraded applicants with graded applicants in the initial application screening process when determining which applicants to invite for interviews (Reference 16). At least one program asks applicants from nongraded programs for a letter of recommendation that comments on the applicant's academic ability (Reference 17). Another program suggests that any residency applicant, whether from a graded or nongraded program, can include a brief discussion about his or her academic performance and learning in his or her letter of intent (Reference 18).

*Make Your Nongraded Transcript Residency Application Stand Out*
Although there seems to be no standard method in residency programs by which to evaluate nongraded transcripts, I believe that applicants from nongraded schools can distinguish their applications from their graded competition in ways that will attract positive attention from residency programs. One way of doing this is to maintain a portfolio of some kind. You may already have a portfolio because many pharmacy schools require them. If you have a portfolio from pharmacy school, you will likely want to modify it before showing it to residency directors. I would focus on a subset of items that would bring significant parts of your curriculum vitae (CV) "to life" as well as demonstrate the type of person you are and why you will make a great resident! You could provide details about the following (not necessarily in this order):

- Significant experiences that have helped develop your character and work ethic
- Significant experiences that have developed your skills and abilities to practice pharmacy and take care of patients
- Significant projects you've completed (individually and with others)
- Significant experiences that you have participated in/led/coordinated
- Honors and achievements (without sounding pretentious!)
- Other items of note that you think set you apart from other applicants

I personally prefer some kind of Web-based, easily navigable portfolio so that residency directors don't have more paper to handle—they can click away at their leisure if they so choose. This might also allow you to embed some video (such as from a presentation you made) that could help them "see you" and get to know you better before and after an interview. You could provide the link to your portfolio on your CV or other appropriate place in the application.

In sum, if you don't have a traditional graded transcript as part of your residency applications, find other ways to make yourself stand out—such as through a portfolio, a letter of intent, and other approaches mentioned in this book. Don't let a nontraditional transcript hold you back from pursuing your top residencies!

## THE REAL REASONS YOU SHOULD LEARN AS MUCH AS YOU CAN (AND GET HIGH GRADES IN THE PROCESS!)

We know that there isn't necessarily strong evidence to support a connection between good grades and having a successful practice, getting a residency, or even learning. There also seems to be an element of "subjectivity" to the very concept of grades. So why would you still want to do your best academically? Beyond the reasons already discussed, such as how your grades can serve as a reflection of your character and priorities, there are other important reasons you should strive to learn as much as you can and do your best academically.

- **Optimal patient care and safety**—Ideally, if you know how to be a good pharmacist and can apply most, if not all, of what you learned in school and experiential training, you should be a valuable resource to your patients, other health care providers, and the health care system. Learning as much as you can is really an issue about patient care and professionalism—putting others' needs above your own. This might be a foreign concept to those who feel that pharmacy school is like many other school experiences, where good grades can mean rewards, scholarships, financial aid, dean's list, and other, more tangible factors. But in the professional world, where one of the hallmarks of being a professional is being competent, learning can take on a deeper meaning. It can mean the difference between recommending a dose that is harmful versus one that is helpful. Learning at the doctoral level takes on a much higher purpose and meaning. It's not about you anymore; it's about those you serve.
- **Credibility and trust**—Your patients and future fellow health care providers will likely not have read your CV or have any idea of your graduating GPA. Instead, they will judge you by your interactions with them—your professionalism, communication style, competence, confidence, and many other factors. Learning

as much as you can (in and outside school) will serve to enhance these characteristics. Grades in and of themselves can do little to enhance your credibility and trust with those who know about your grades. However, at the end of the day, it comes down to how you treat people and how well you do your job.

- **Personal satisfaction, confidence, and the challenge of achieving your goals**—

    *If there is no struggle, there is no progress.*

    —Frederick Douglass

    Doing well academically can be incredibly satisfying—you have worked hard in your studies to achieve your potential. You have likely sacrificed time with family and friends, or time for yourself. You have had to exercise discipline to focus and stick to your goals. It feels good to be rewarded for this hard work by good grades and to know that others have recognized those achievements! High marks can also help you feel confident in your knowledge base to practice. Granted, most of us don't ever feel completely confident going into our APPEs, or on that first day of practice with your new pharmacy license ("how will I ever remember everything???"), but it certainly doesn't hurt your confidence if you know you did your best academically and learned as much as you could. Especially if your focus was on learning and developing into a competent professional.

- **Preparation for residency**—I have already stated that learning as much as you can while in school should help prepare you for a residency, together with following the advice of the other chapters in this book. It also seems that in the competitive residency application environment, achievement of good grades will help you be invited to interview. When all is said and done, if your good grades reflect that you have learned a great deal, then you should be better prepared to succeed in a residency than if your grades were not so stellar.

## CONCLUSION—THE BALANCE

Each chapter in this book talks about a different aspect of your pharmacy school career in which you should gain experience and do well. One question you may be asking yourself is, "How can I possibly do all of these things and still spend much of my time studying and learning for understanding?" I can't emphasize enough the importance of trying to balance priorities in the achievement of goals. Because many of us may not naturally know how to do this well, I am a strong advocate of seeking assistance. The right books, Web sites, classes, and people can serve as helpful resources in achieving your goals. The office of student affairs at your school likely has resources to help you in this endeavor. There is also a book chapter on time management written specifically for pharmacy students that might offer you wisdom (Reference 19). Finding upper-class student mentors can also help you along this journey. Seek out the students who are both involved in a variety of school activities and who do well academically. If you are not aware of who those students might be, check the Rho Chi membership, or ask your faculty or staff in the office of student affairs about students who would be good mentors/role models for residency preparation. Perhaps you have the luxury of interacting with pharmacy residents either in your practice or the classroom. You should ask their advice for how you can best prepare for residency. When establishing priorities during pharmacy school about how you are going to accomplish all of your goals, you should consider your learning above all else, for all the reasons previously described. After all, if you don't "make the grade," you won't even have the opportunity to become a pharmacist in the first place!

In conclusion, grades are certainly not the "end-all, be-all" for whether you are selected for a residency. But they can be an influential factor in that decision-making process, for all the reasons noted in this chapter. What matters most is that you take advantage of this amazing opportunity called pharmacy school to learn as much as you can so that you will be a valuable service to your patients and society. It is also incredibly important for your well-being to make sure you balance your priorities in a way that helps you achieve your goals but is not detrimental to your physical, mental, and emotional health. Best of luck to you in your career!

## REFERENCES

1. Knowles MS. Self-Directed Learning: A Guide for Learners and Teachers. Englewood Cliffs, NJ: Prentice Hall/Cambridge, 1975.
2. Rouse MJ. Continuing professional development in pharmacy. Am J Health Syst Pharm 2004;61:2069-76.
3. Accreditation Council for Pharmacy Education. Continuing Professional Development. Chicago: Accreditation Council for Pharmacy Education. Available at https://www.acpe-accredit.org/ceproviders/CPD.asp. Accessed September 11, 2012.
4. O'Brocta R, Abu-Baker A, Budukh P, Gandhi M, Lavigne J, Birnie C. A continuous professional development process for first-year pharmacy students. Am J Pharm Educ 2012;76:Article 29.
5. Erickson BL, Strommer DW. Teaching College Freshmen. San Francisco: Jossey-Bass, 1991.
6. Walvoord BE, Anderson VJ. Chapter 1. The power of grading for learning and assessment. In: Walvoord BE, Anderson VJ, eds. Effective Grading: A Tool for Learning and Assessment. San Francisco: Jossey-Bass, 1998:2.
7. Kidd RS, Latif DA. Traditional and novel predictors of classroom and clerkship success of pharmacy students. Am J Pharm Educ 2003;67:Article 109.
8. Allen DD, Bond CA. Prepharmacy indicators of success in pharmacy school: grade point averages, pharmacy college ad-mission test, communication abilities, and critical thinking skills. Pharmacotherapy 2001;21:842-9.
9. Guskey TR, Pollio HR. Grading Systems – School, Higher Education. Education Encyclopedia – StateUniversity.com. Available at http://education.stateuniversity.com/pages/2017/Grading-Systems.html. Accessed September 19, 2012.
10. Jellenick-Cohen SP, Cohen V, Bucher KL, Likourezos A. Factors used by pharmacy residency programs to select residents. Am J Health Syst Pharm 2012;69:1105-8.
11. Mancuso CE, Paloucek FP. Understanding and preparing for pharmacy practice residency interviews. Am J Health Syst Pharm 2004;61:1686-9.
12. McCollum M, Hansen LB. Characteristics of doctor of pharmacy graduates entering and not entering residency training upon graduation. Am J Pharm Educ 2005;69:Article 42.
13. Caballero J, Benavides S, Steinberg JG, et al. Development of a residency interviewing preparatory seminar. Am J Health Syst Pharm 2012;69:400-4.
14. Proceedings of the 2008 ASHP National Residency Preceptors Conference. Am J Health Syst Pharm 2009;66:e53-4.
15. Jungnickel PW. Grade-point averages and class rankings in evaluation of pharmacy residency applicants. Am J Health Syst Pharm 2010;67:1500, 1502.
16. P. Scheele, personal communication, August 2012.
17. Anonymous, personal communication, August 2012.
18. Paloucek FP. Better letter of intent for pharmacy residency applications. Am J Health Syst Pharm 2011;68:2218.
19. Hammer DP. Time management/organizational skills. In: Desselle S, Zgarrick D, eds. Pharmacy Management, 3rd ed. New York: McGraw-Hill, 2012:153-73.

# STEP III
# GET INVOLVED

Janet P. Engle, Pharm.D., FAPhA

## INTRODUCTION

Pharmacy school can be overwhelming. Heavy course loads and studying can take up much of your time each day. Of importance, however, is designating time for a vital activity of your professional future: getting involved! Although doing well in school is important, it is also critical to set time aside to get involved in professional and community activities. Even though networking and becoming active in outside professional activities require time you may feel you don't have, it is valuable to apply your knowledge and learning from others outside your time in the classroom.

Getting involved can encompass many things. It does not necessarily mean you have to run for president of a student branch of a professional association. Participating in student organization committees and community health screenings, organizing a fundraiser or social event, and participating in a state legislative day are all examples of getting involved. Many students don't realize the importance of this until later in their studies or after they graduate. By then, valuable time has been lost in best preparing to be a standout residency candidate.

## WHY GET INVOLVED?

You will reap many personal and professional benefits from getting involved in your profession and community. From defining your career goals to developing valuable leadership skills—all will improve your chances of acquiring a residency position upon graduation.

Leadership is an expected outcome for American Society of Health-System Pharmacists (ASHP)-accredited postgraduate year one (PGY1) residency programs. By already having some leadership activities and professional involvement as a student, you will be better prepared to take on the rigors of a residency and, as such, will stand out from other candidates. Learning to be an effective pharmacist does not occur solely from going to class, highlighting your notes, transcribing them onto study sheets, and studying. The most competitive residency applicants will have engaged in a variety of activities outside class work during their time in pharmacy school.

For students interested in pursuing residency training, getting involved is not optional. Professional involvement by a student indicates that the student can multitask and understand the benefits of giving back to the profession of pharmacy by participating in professional and community activities. It is important and ultimately rewarding to give back to the profession through your involvement in pharmacy associations and pharmacy-related community activities. As a pharmacy student, you can use your skills and perspective to enhance and advance our profession. Even as a student, your involvement provides an opportunity to directly affect the profession. Becoming involved in professional associations affords you the ability to shape policy and voice your opinions, which in turn can help shape practice in the way you would like to see it evolve. Providing pharmacy-related services in the community familiarizes the public with the role of the pharmacist and allows you to gain practical experience working with patients.

Many advantages of participating in professional associations and community activities exist in addition to developing leadership abilities and helping shape the profession. For instance, you may be unfamiliar with some of the issues affecting the profession as a student, especially in the early years of the curriculum, but becoming involved in an association can broaden your perspective on international, national, state, and local issues affecting pharmacy and health care. Even as a student, you should be knowledgeable about current issues facing the profession, including the role of the pharmacist in patient care. Having an understanding of current affairs related to pharmacy will help you in your studies and make you a more competitive residency candidate. During your interview, you will have an understanding of a wide range of topics that you can discuss with the interviewer, which will set you apart from other candidates, who may not be as knowledgeable.

Another advantage to joining a professional association is gaining access to the organization's membership benefits. Each organization has publications, some of which are targeted directly to students. For a very small investment in time, you can read these publications and keep abreast of issues facing the profession and health care in general. You may also receive student discounts on meetings, publications, and other materials offered by the association. Many student organizations will routinely hold information sessions about residency opportunities and the skills needed to secure a residency such as how to build your curriculum vitae (CV) and improve your interviewing skills.

Getting involved in organizations that emphasize patient care and clinical pharmacy can help you more accurately focus your career goals and assist you in determining the attributes that a PGY1 residency should have to meet your needs. By being active in outside organizations throughout your pharmacy curriculum, you will have a better sense of what type of program may meet your needs. Involvement in local or state organizations may afford you opportunities to network with the residency directors of the programs that most interest you. When the time comes to interview, you will have an advantage over other candidates because you will already be known to the program, and you will be able to intelligently discuss a variety of topics related to current events in pharmacy.

Finally, participating in professional or community activities will afford you the ability to meet and work with colleagues you would not normally have been able to collaborate with, thereby expanding your network. In the early years of pharmacy school, involvement may result from asking an upperclassman with similar interests and the desire to pursue a residency to serve as a mentor. As that person progresses through the curriculum and ultimately secures a residency, you can learn from his or her journey. In addition, problem solving may become easier as you interact and brainstorm with a wider group of colleagues. Getting involved can help keep you excited about the profession and provide another forum for pharmacy-related activities that can help you not only obtain a residency position, but also enhance your career as a pharmacist.

> *As a pharmacy student, I wish I had run for a national position in a professional organization. These positions open up a number of networking opportunities and provide you with a great leadership experience.*
>
> —Kathleen Lusk, 2011/12 PGY2 Internal Medicine Resident at St. Luke's Hospital, in Chesterfield, Mo.

Keep in mind that balance is important as you prepare to be an excellent residency candidate. Residency program directors look for well-rounded candidates who display the ability to multitask. Besides doing well in coursework, you will find it helpful to show that you were able to participate successfully in extracurricular activities, together with other obligations like service activities and part-time employment.

In addition to your extracurricular and community activities, try to find time for other activities you enjoy (e.g., participating in sports, working out) or hobbies (e.g., gardening, photography, music, sewing, cooking, woodworking). Making time for your hobbies and social life will contribute to your overall well-being and produce a well-rounded residency candidate.

## OPTIONS FOR INVOLVEMENT IN PROFESSIONAL ORGANIZATIONS

There are many pharmacy-related organizations to consider for involvement. Most residency directors will review your CV, looking for a several different activities that show leadership. Keep in mind that an activity valued by one residency program may not be valued by another, so it is advisable to be involved in several types of organizations. Involvement in organizations or projects unrelated to pharmacy is also an option. Although it is not recommended to focus completely on non-pharmacy-related undertakings, it is reasonable to include some of these activities throughout your time in pharmacy school if they interest you. Non-pharmacy-related involvement should also be included on your CV.

It is never too early to become active in pharmacy, interprofessional, and community organizations. To get the most from your time in pharmacy school, consider putting together a written plan outlining the groups you wish to become involved with, potential activities or committees to work on, and, finally, potential leadership positions you may wish to pursue. As you think through your plan for involvement, take on responsibility in incremental steps. You do not have to do everything in 1 year. Table 1 outlines the types of activities to consider during each year of the curriculum. If the task seems overwhelming, enlist the aid of an upperclassman who has been active in student organizations or the faculty adviser of one of the groups. Writing down your ideas and revisiting them once or twice a year will help you stay focused and not let opportunities go by because you are too bogged down with schoolwork to properly plan for your extracurricular activities.

As you participate in various activities, be sure to document them on your CV or in a portfolio. If you wait until the end of the year or until you start interviewing, you are likely to forget some of them. If you have been particularly involved in a project, save some examples of flyers or photos from the event to place in your portfolio. Be sure to highlight your productivity, whether it is committee work, an elected position, or general membership activities. You may also want to include information about any part-time jobs you may have, the number of hours worked, and any leadership or special projects that you took on in your position.

When seeking to get involved in activities such as pharmacy organizations, community organizations, interprofessional groups, or professional fraternities, think about your interests and any possible constraints on your participation. Although you may be interested in international pharmacy, you may not have the resources or time to attend meetings or become involved in a meaningful way; in this case, it may be better to initially choose a student organization where you are more likely to attend meetings and participate. Thus, begin looking for an organization that closely meets your practice interests. Consider organizations with broad or interprofessional memberships as well as specialty organizations. Many such organizations will provide meeting programming targeted toward students as well as networking opportunities in which you can take part.

If you are just entering pharmacy school, check your school's Web site to determine the professional student organizations and professional fraternities that are available. If the information is not posted on the Web site, inquire during orientation or contact the student affairs office to discover your options. Table 2 lists some common student organizations and professional fraternities that are present on most campuses. If you are just starting out and are unsure of your specific interests in pharmacy, consider joining a broad-based organization like the American Pharmacists Association Academy of Student Pharmacists (APhA-ASP). As you continue through the pharmacy curriculum, you will develop special interests. If you choose to focus on clinical pharmacy, the American College of Clinical Pharmacy (ACCP) may best represent your interests. Most schools also have student chapters of some of the more focused organizations such as ASHP or the National Community Pharmacists Association. As you begin to define and narrow your career goals, it is acceptable to discontinue your involvement in one organization to become more involved in another. Determine the number of organizations you can afford to maintain membership in, and pursue activities and leadership opportunities in those that best meet your needs and provide the types of programs and events you want to be involved in.

In addition to the large national and international organizations and fraternities, state and local associations have opportunities for student involvement. For example, most states have a pharmacy association that represents all practice sites and a health-system association that

**Table 1.** Navigating Getting Involved by Year in the Curriculum

| Professional Year | Recommended Activities |
|---|---|
| P1 | • Join at least one broad-based non-specialty student branch of pharmacy organizations on campus.<br>• Attend general meetings on a regular basis.<br>• Explore ways of getting involved—does not have to be in a leadership position.<br>• Attend a local or state pharmacy meeting. |
| P2 | • Continue work with organization from P1 year.<br>• If a particular specialty is of interest, consider joining a specialty organization or a professional fraternity.<br>• Continue committee work; consider chairing a committee or pursuing an elected position.<br>• Explore opportunities to participate in community or interprofessional activities possibly related to one of the professional organizations you belong to.<br>• Attend a local or state pharmacy meeting—look for opportunities to get involved; check for a mentoring program.<br>• If you don't have work experience in a pharmacy, find some shadowing opportunities to increase your familiarity with practice in a variety of settings.<br>• Consider attending a regional meeting such as the APhA-ASP Midyear Regional Meeting or a national meeting such as the ASHP Midyear Clinical Meeting, ACCP Annual Meeting, or the APhA Annual Meeting.[a]<br>• As you do these activities, document them on your CV or in your portfolio. |

| Professional Year | Recommended Activities |
| --- | --- |
| P3 | - Continue work with organizations of choice.
- Pursue an elected leadership position.
- Continue work on community and interprofessional activities such as health fairs and screenings.
- If service learning is available at your school, participate in a service learning project.
- Attend a local or state pharmacy meeting—look for opportunities to get involved.
- Continue to find some shadowing opportunities to increase your familiarity with practice in a variety of settings if you haven't already done so.
- Attend the ASHP Midyear Clinical Meeting to get familiar with the residency recruiting process; attend Residency Showcase.
- As you do these activities, document them on your CV or in your portfolio. |
| P4 | - Continue work with organizations of choice.
- Continue committee work if possible with clerkship schedule.
- Continue work on community or interprofessional activities such as health fairs and screenings.
- Attend ASHP Midyear Clinical Meeting; enroll in Personnel Placement Service, attend Residency Showcase.
- As you do these activities, document them on your CV or in your portfolio. |

[a]Reference 1.
ACCP = American College of Clinical Pharmacy; APhA = American Pharmacists Association; ASHP = American Society of Health-System Pharmacists; ASP = Academy of Student Pharmacists; CV = curriculum vitae.

represents pharmacists in health-system pharmacy practice. In some states (e.g., Iowa, Wisconsin), these associations have merged, with one association representing both groups. Many state associations have formal mentoring programs in which a student pharmacist can sign up to work with a pharmacist-mentor. Attending these programs can be an excellent way to meet leaders in the profession as well as residency directors and get their advice on your career path. Even if your state does not have a formal mentoring program, getting involved on a local and state level will allow you to network with local pharmacists as well as residency directors. This is an excellent opportunity to get to know these individuals outside the residency interview arena.

As you move through the professional curriculum, you will want to be sure to incorporate the activities and grade point requirements needed to be considered for induction into the honor and leadership societies, Rho Chi and Phi Lambda Sigma. Most pharmacy schools have chapters of these honor societies, and the chapter advisers can assist you with the requirements for being considered for induction. Information about these societies can also be found on the Web sites listed in Table 2. Being inducted into one or both of these societies shows the attainment of excellent grades, in Rho Chi, and excellent grades and leadership abilities, in Phi Lambda Sigma.

## HOW TO GET INVOLVED?

Once you have an idea of the student organizations at your school, you can start planning a strategy to get involved. As a first-year student, start attending the general meetings of the organization. Get an idea of the activities involved in by the group. Explore possible committees that might be of interest to you. Possibly volunteer for a small activity just to get your feet wet. Even participating in one or two small activities during the first semester can help in your quest to obtain a residency. The more people you get to know, the wider your circle of colleagues becomes. You never know when one or more of these people can help you later in your career.

If you do not have a student chapter of an organization you are interested in or if you wish to get involved in the local or state affiliates of a pharmacy organization, you can begin by perusing the Web sites of these organizations to discover the opportunities available for students. You can also attend the general meetings. Even if you do not volunteer for committees or other activities, you will benefit from networking and meeting practitioners in your area. Look for opportunities to attend social events such as alumni and state pharmacy association receptions.

These are great ways to become acquainted with people and network. You may also be able to learn about additional opportunities for getting involved at these functions.

Consider joining pharmacy-related online social networking groups. This is an easy way to stay informed and participate in discussions about issues important to pharmacy, and involvement in these groups does not require a large time or financial commitment. For example, both APhA and ASHP have active Facebook pages that are updated on a regular basis. Both organizations are also active on Twitter. You do not have to be a member of these organizations to participate in their social networking sites.

Participate whenever possible, whether on a committee that matches your interests or simply in a discussion at one of the gatherings. Make it known that you are willing to become more involved. Once you commit to a particular task, actively participate, follow through, and meet deadlines. Nothing is worse than volunteering for something and then not doing it well or at all. People remember this lack of follow-through, which can impede your advancement later, so be sure to strive for excellence and see your tasks to completion.

Look for mentor-faculty who have successfully achieved leadership positions in pharmacy organizations, and obtain their advice on how best to get involved and reach your ultimate goal of obtaining a residency position. Every association has its own organizational culture, and receiving advice from someone knowledgeable about the culture can help. Start small during your first year of school, and add additional responsibilities as you progress through the curriculum. If you take a focused, stepwise approach, being involved won't overwhelm you, and the rewards later in your career can be huge.

As a student, you may wonder whether it is worth your very limited time to attend a professional local, state, or national meeting that may require travel time and a day or more away from school. Nevertheless, the benefits to attending professional meetings are many, whether they are student meetings on campus or local, state, or national meetings that last 1 or more days. For example, meeting attendance allows you to learn about new developments in pharmacy, expand your knowledge in an area of interest, view the newest products if there is an exhibit hall, build and enlarge your network of contacts, and discover residency opportunities. Taking a break from your normal routine can be not only educational, but also reenergizing.

To get the most from attending any professional meeting, prepare for it. If you are attending a local or on-campus meeting, try to learn who usually attends and determine with whom you would like to

**Table 2.** List of Selected National Pharmacy Organizations, Fraternities, and Honor Societies with Student Opportunities for Involvement

| Organization/Web Site | Focus | Some Potential Areas of Involvement for Students |
|---|---|---|
| Academy of Managed Care Pharmacy (AMCP) amcp.org | Represents pharmacists who practice in managed health care environments | National: student pharmacist committee; student programming at meetings<br><br>School chapter: officer, committee chair, committee member; participate in Pharmacy and Therapeutics (P&T) competition |
| American College of Clinical Pharmacy (ACCP) accp.com | Represents clinical pharmacists, scientists, educators, administrators, students, residents, and fellows dedicated to excellence in clinical pharmacy | National: participate in Student Advisory Committee, submit articles for StuNews,[a] participate in practice and research networks (PRNs) or ACCP Advocates Program<br><br>School: volunteer as your school's pharmacy student liaison, participate in the Clinical Pharmacy Challenge student team competition |
| American Pharmacists Association (APhA) Pharmacist.com | The national professional society of pharmacists representing pharmacists in all practice settings | National: elected positions for students at the national and regional levels, participate in committees, attend regional midyear meetings, participate in student programming at the annual meeting, participate in the APhA Leadership Training Series<br><br>School chapter: (Academy of Student Pharmacists – ASP); elected office, committee chairs, committee membership, participate in a variety of patient care projects (e.g., Operation Immunization); participate in the Patient Counseling Competition |
| American Society of Health-System Pharmacists (ASHP) ASHP.org | Represents pharmacists who practice in hospitals, health maintenance organizations, long-term care facilities, home care, and other components of health care systems | National: automatically enrolled in the Pharmacy Student Forum, can serve as an appointed leader in the forum, opportunities for committee and advisory group participation<br><br>Student Society: elected office, committee chairs, committee membership, participate in chapter projects, participate in the Clinical Skills Competition |

| Organization/Web Site | Focus | Some Potential Areas of Involvement for Students |
|---|---|---|
| National Community Pharmacists Association (NCPA) ncpanet.org | Represents pharmacy owners, managers, and employees of independent community pharmacies | National: can be appointed to the National Student Leadership Council or steering committee, student programming at annual convention Student Chapter: elected office, committee chairs, committee membership, participate in chapter projects |
| Phi Lambda Sigma philambdasigma.org | The national pharmacy leadership society | Must meet qualifications to be inducted into the society. General requirements can be found on the Web site; each chapter may have additional requirements. Student Chapter: elected office, committee chairs, committee membership, participation in chapter projects |
| Rho Chi Society rhochi.org | The academic honor society in pharmacy | Must meet qualifications to be inducted into the society. General requirements can be found on the Web site; each chapter may have additional requirements. Student Chapter: elected office, committee chairs, committee membership, participation in chapter projects |
| Professional pharmacy fraternities; some examples include Alpha Zeta Omega (alphazetaomega.net), Kappa Epsilon (kappaepsilon.org), Kappa Psi (kappapsi.org), Lambda Kappa Sigma (LKS.org), and Phi Delta Chi (phideltachi.org) | Professional pharmacy fraternities that focus on promoting the profession of pharmacy and leadership | Student Chapter: elected office, committee chairs, committee membership, participation in chapter projects |

[a]Reference 2.
Note: All listed organizations provide reduced dues for students.

make contact. It could be an excellent opportunity to get to know the faculty adviser for that organization, for example, on a personal basis. For larger state and national meetings, access the program (usually published on the meeting Web site) before leaving for it, and make a schedule of the sessions that are of most interest to you. Determine whether there are any special sessions or tracks for pharmacy students, and take advantage of them. If you are close to seeking a residency position, familiarize yourself with the various resources offered at the conference. Informal networking may be just as effective as a formal residency interview.

Taking the time to plan ahead to get the most from a professional meeting, whether it occurs on campus, in your town, or across the country, will help ensure that your meeting participation contributes to your professional development and the likelihood of getting that coveted residency position.

## GETTING INVOLVED IN THE COMMUNITY

Students have many opportunities to get involved in the community. Many of the student pharmacy organizations organize events such as blood pressure screenings, poison prevention activities, brown bag medication reviews, and immunization fairs. Most APhA-ASP chapters participate in patient care projects such as Operation Immunization that specifically target outreach to the community. Many times, health fairs are looking for pharmacists and pharmacy students to set up a table and provide education. If your pharmacy school is not associated with a medical center that is involved in health fairs, contact the department of pharmacy in a hospital or a community pharmacy in your town to volunteer your time in health fairs and other outreach activities they may be organizing. Another option is to organize a pharmacy-themed community event yourself such as a brown bag medication review with a church, gym, or other local businesses. Develop a plan for the event, ensuring that you have sufficient volunteer support from other pharmacy students and faculty and remembering that you should have a licensed pharmacist with you at all times to supervise community activities. Contact the church or business and present your plan, asking for the support you need, whether it is space, marketing assistance, or financial support for supplies.

As a student, you should make time to get involved in this type of undertaking. In addition to the activity's looking good on your CV, you will have the opportunity to practice the skills you are learning in pharmacy school in a real-life setting. By participating in these types of events, you will be setting yourself up to be a standout residency candidate. In addition, your involvement in the community helps promote the profession of pharmacy and the expertise of the pharmacist to the public and to other health care professionals you may be working with.

## SERVICE LEARNING AND SELF-REFLECTION

Service learning combines learning with providing service. Students participate in an organized service activity with educational objectives that meet community needs. If your pharmacy program offers service learning as an option, take advantage of it. Service learning helps the student connect theory that he or she learns in the pharmacy curriculum with practice in a real-world setting. In service learning, the student and the community benefit. A self-reflection is usually a component of the experience, such that you will have an opportunity to employ critical thinking and place your role as a pharmacist in a larger context. In general, you will be asked to reflect on the service you provided, what you learned, what your thoughts are on issues raised by the activity, and your successes or problems. You may be asked to keep a journal that may be reviewed by a faculty member. Self-reflection activities may include describing an event that occurred during service in which you may not have known how to react or what to say and, in retrospect, describing several scenarios that you could have used to address the problem. Other forms of reflection could take place in a discussion board for the class online or in formal responses to predetermined questions for the experience.

## FINAL WORDS

Although the goal of this chapter has been to outline why getting involved is important to your career and viability as a standout residency candidate, there are some words of caution. *Pharmacy is a small world*; therefore…

- Don't overcommit yourself. Volunteer to do only what is reasonable. There is nothing worse than having an organization or individuals counting on you and not meeting the deadlines or delivering the end product. Pharmacy is a small world, and word will get around if your commitments aren't met.
- Don't bad-mouth your employer, preceptor, other students, faculty, or anyone else. You never know when the person about whom you are saying less-than-complimentary things can become your boss or become involved with a decision related to hiring you or granting you an award. Also, don't say derogatory things about

other schools, residency programs, or career choices that may be different from yours. It pays to be positive. Avoid burning bridges because you never know when you will need to cross them in the future.

## CONCLUSION

Getting involved in professional organizations and other activities outside the pharmacy curriculum is essential to securing a residency position. It is also critical for a successful career in pharmacy and is a wonderful opportunity to give back to the profession and help drive it forward. Learning to be a successful practitioner does not occur in a vacuum. Participating in the profession, community activities, and service learning affords you the opportunity to apply the knowledge and skills you have learned in the pharmacy curriculum. These vital skills, although important in helping you obtain a residency position, will serve you well throughout your career.

## REFERENCES

1. Pharmacist.com [homepage on the Internet]. APhA-ASP Leadership Training Series. Washington, DC: American Pharmacists Association. Available at www.pharmacist.com/Content/NavigationMenu2/LeadershipProfessionalism/LeadershipTrainingSeries/default.htm. Accessed June 26, 2012.
2. ACCP.com [homepage on the Internet]. StuNet News. Lenexa, KS: American College of Clinical Pharmacy. Available at www.accp.com/stunet/newsletter.aspx. Accessed June 26, 2012.

# STEP IV

# DEVELOP LEADERSHIP AND MANAGEMENT ABILITIES

Donald E. Letendre, Pharm.D.; and Brandon J. Patterson, Pharm.D.

## CHAPTER SUMMARY

When selecting a resident, pharmacy preceptors and residency program directors look for candidates who possess an aptitude for leadership and management. This chapter will help you, through self-reflection, determine some steps you can take as a student to help hone your leadership and management skills. In addition, this chapter will provide strategies and tactics for time and project management.

The world is teeming with writings that address the broad topics of leadership and management. In a guide such as this, it would be a disservice to you to distill so much of what has been written into a so-called formula for success. Rather, in the pages that follow, we hope you will find some useful kernels of advice that have been derived from years of engagement with students and residents.

In a world of perpetual change, especially in the area of health care, there is a constant need for "change agents." We are certain that on many occasions, you have heard refrains from faculty and preceptors that resemble the following:

> As students, you should feel fortunate. In my day, pharmacy was practiced very differently with limited interaction with patients, and the scope of technical support paled in comparison to what exists today.

Indeed, the practice of pharmacy and the support systems that have evolved are vastly different from those of just a few decades ago. But changes did not just happen without forethought and purpose. Countless individuals exercised the leadership and management skills necessary to make those changes possible. Collectively, they can be described as our profession's change agents.

It is important to stress "collectively." Too often, students hold the perception that their contributions must be of a magnitude to warrant special recognition by being out front and leading the charge. Although it is true that many individuals are credited with new concepts that brought about meaningful change (referred to as "Big L" later in the chapter), virtually none of these changes would have been possible without the contributions of thousands of "little l's" (discussed later in the chapter, but essentially, those who exhibit leadership without having authority defined by a position or title) whose influence and leadership helped implement and refine the ideas of others into the models of practice we witness today.

Where did these change agents come from? It could easily be debated, particularly in the practice of health-systems pharmacy and clinical education, that a vast number of these individuals are the product of residency training. And similar champions of change are emerging in other segments of the profession (e.g., community care and emerging specialties) as residency training branches out into those areas. It should come as no surprise, then, that residency program directors have long sought out candidates who show leadership and management abilities, knowing full well that their progeny are tomorrow's change agents, both Big L's and little l's.

## LEADERSHIP

L.P. is a 23-year-old Pharm.D. student in the second professional year of her 4-year Pharm.D. program at the University of Iowa. She has a 3.2/4.0 GPA and is considering residency training. She is worried that her grades will not be strong enough to land her the residency she desires, but she has a passion for helping patients. She wants to translate that passion into leadership opportunities that can set her apart from other residency candidates. She has tried running for elected office in the school chapter of her favorite professional association but has been unsuccessful in her bids so far. What can L.P. do to fulfill her desire to be a leader? How can L.P. develop and hone leadership skills in the next few years?

In laying the foundation for leadership, it is important to recognize early on that acquiring leadership traits takes time and does not suddenly manifest itself overnight, thus limiting the notion that leaders are "born" (Reference 1). Much like a child must learn how to walk before running, so too must an emerging leader learn the precepts of leadership one step at a time. It is only through life's experiences as a well as through a series of exercises and tasks that an individual develops the qualities of leadership and gains the confidence and experience to lead.

Observationally, it would appear that most humans want to be led rather than lead. Think about it ... there is a high degree of probability that you can readily identify individuals who consistently step forward when it comes time to lead. Hopefully, you are among those who have done so. If so, then you understand firsthand the importance of "ownership" ... ownership of whatever it is that you were leading. In taking ownership, you exercise responsibility, and through your responsibility, you convey a willingness to be held accountable for the actions you take as the leader.

For example, consider something as simple as a school project that involved a few of your classmates or something far more complex like an organization you were asked or elected to lead. In either case, taking ownership was critical to success. And when you took ownership, you exercised responsibility and demonstrated many other skills that represented leadership including, but certainly not limited to, team-building, articulation of a vision or plan, delegation, communication, and confidence. Together, these actions and attitudes would likely have resulted in others on your team identifying you as a leader. And in doing so, you were being held accountable by those you were leading, whether expressly stated or not.

Moreover, opportunities to lead should be viewed as a sacred privilege. After all, if exercised properly, you will change others' lives through their acceptance of the path or plan you have laid out. Also, without their participation, you have no one to lead. It is imperative to always remember that those around you represent your potential team. In considering this point, it is worth noting the old adage that "with great authority comes great responsibility." As a leader, you will have no greater responsibility than to the members of your team.

One noteworthy event that captures the essence of this principle can be found in Lansing's book *Endurance*, the superbly narrated account of Ernest Shackleton's 1915–1916 failed attempt to cross Antarctica and the astonishing journey that followed in which he miraculously led all of his 27 men safely back home (Reference 2). Through perseverance, a keen understanding of their environment, superb navigational skills, and the attributes noted earlier … team-building, articulation of a vision or plan, delegation, communication, and confidence …, Shackleton showed tremendous leadership and earned the respect of his men. In the book, Lansing notes that Shackleton came to be addressed by his men simply as "Boss."

> It had a pleasant ring of familiarity about it, but at the same time "Boss" had the connotation of absolute authority. It was therefore particularly apt, and exactly fitted Shackleton's outlook and behavior…. [He] was simply emotionally incapable of forgetting—even for an instant—his position and the responsibility it entailed. The [27] others might rest, or find escape by the device of living for the moment. But for Shackleton there was little rest and no escape. The responsibility was entirely his, and a man could not be in his presence without feeling this.

As you begin to explore residencies, it is helpful to gain a greater understanding—and regularly remind yourself—of some of the basic principles of leadership … responsibility, perseverance, accountability, team-building, articulation of a vision or plan, delegation, communication, and confidence, among others. Although many of these qualities may seem self-evident, they are often misunderstood or made out to be unattainable. Make no mistake; there is a leader within you, and at different times throughout your career, you will have the opportunity to be either a Big L or little l, as noted in the section that follows.

Therefore, the question isn't its existence; rather, the question is, as a student and in the formative years of your career like "L.P."—the second-year pharmacy student noted at the beginning of this section—will you take the initiative, if you haven't already done so, to bring your skills to the surface? Grades are not the sole factor by which you will be evaluated as a candidate for residency training. Remember, people, for the most part, want to be led. Residency program directors are looking for evidence of your leadership. Leadership is what our profession needs, and serving as a leader will bring you an immense degree of personal and professional satisfaction as well as gain the attention of those considering you for a residency.

## Big L vs. little l Leaders

One common misconception of leadership is that leaders must hold a position of great authority, like a CEO, dean, director of pharmacy, or national president of a student organization. Being bestowed vast amounts of authority is not a requirement for being a leader!

Positional leaders, like those mentioned earlier, are considered Big L leaders. People who exhibit leadership without having authority defined by a position are little l leaders (Reference 3). True leaders are masters of exercising power within the confines of authority granted or obtained, irrespective of the situation, regardless of being a Big L or little l leader. In this respect, students seldom recognize the level of authority they can exercise and the attendant responsibility that follows … in the classroom, the college, their community, and their personal lives.

So, how do you exhibit leadership without a given position? To answer this question, it is best to think about leadership in its most fundamental form. Leadership is a process of influencing others to achieve a desired outcome. When viewed through this lens, leadership opportunities are abundant. Helping your classmates succeed in the curriculum, providing services to people with needs in your community, and stepping up to the plate and committing yourself to making your surroundings better are all ways to show leadership.

It is helpful to remember that leadership often requires a high degree of self-initiative, even when someone may have been thrust into a leadership role. When given or taking the opportunity to lead, whether you are in a Big L role or serving as a little l, it is imperative that you take the initiative to exercise the basic precepts of leadership noted earlier. In all likelihood, you have already heard the term *self-starter*. Leaders don't wait for things to happen; rather, through leadership, they make things happen. They have self-initiative; they are self-starters. Residency program directors will seek candidates who possess this skill, knowing full well that candidates who become the best residents are often those who showed self-initiative as a student because this trait is fundamental to good leadership.

**Leadership Philosophy**

Without a leadership philosophy, you cannot lead. Others look to your leadership philosophy to decide whether to follow you. A leadership philosophy is nothing more than what you believe in regarding your role as leader. As innocuous as that definition seems, many people do not see themselves as a leader and thus never take time to establish their leadership philosophy. Do not make this mistake. A leadership philosophy may be simple. For example, a leader may have the philosophy that leaders exist solely for the betterment of their followers. This statement defines the core of what this leader believes, and his or her actions should reflect that belief. Take the time to write down and commit to specific beliefs you have about leadership.

Beliefs that underpin your thoughts about leadership are based in your leadership perspective. The leadership actions you take and the behaviors you display convey to others your leadership perspective. A leadership perspective is the essence of how you engage your followers, and it helps shape your decision-making as a leader—it is how you shape your leadership philosophy. Understanding different perspectives of leadership allows you to use the best one for your leadership needs. It may also help you study the leadership actions of others, an important activity for you to do when developing your own leadership skills.

Because leadership is primarily an influence relationship built on social exchanges, organizational frames is one set of diverse leadership perspectives. There are many other perspectives, but this set has been used by leaders in many disciplines to understand how leaders shape and influence their organizational environment and the people operating within those organizations. The organizational frames approach describes how exchanges of goods and services and development of relationships occur within an organized group of people. Boleman and Deal describe the four organizational frames as structural, human resource, political, and symbolic (Reference 4). Within each frame, leaders have different priorities and use different techniques in providing leadership.

Structural frame leaders concern themselves with maintaining hierarchy and establishing clear sets of rules for team members. They emphasize the creation of a clear vision and mission for their organizations and reward followers on the basis of completing assigned tasks. Human resources frame leaders place emphasis on developing and supporting the humanity of their followers. They develop relationships to overcome conflict and strive to instill in followers a sense of self-accomplishment. Political leaders understand the importance of power in influencing followers and strive to build coalitions within their group and with other external stakeholders. Bargaining and negotiation are primary tactics of the political leader. Finally, symbolic leaders understand the importance of ritual and ceremony. They seek to create memorable moments and articulate messages to advance organizational goals.

Being aware of the four broadly defined leadership perspectives allows you to select the tactics that best fit your needs in completing a leadership task. For example, you may be in a situation where new students are entering the college of pharmacy, and you are helping lead an effort to acclimate them to their new environment. Structurally, you may create a vision about what you wish to accomplish. Thinking like a human resources leader, you may involve your committee in many informal discussions about what will take place at the welcoming event. Politically, you reach out to other student organizations on campus to examine the materials that other groups use to welcome new students to campus. Finally, as a symbolic leader, you will rally the committee by creating a symbol of their efforts, such as a shirt that all volunteers will wear when welcoming the new students. Each perspective provides the leader a path toward action for any situation. Push yourself to think in all four frames each time you serve in a leadership capacity. You will be amazed at how inclusive and comprehensive your actions become.

**Leadership Styles**
When you perform as a leader, you display a particular way of doing things … this is commonly referred to as your leadership style. For many decades, scholars have investigated leadership styles in hopes of finding the "best" one. They have not found it. What is important is that you understand some common leadership behaviors and incorporate a diverse set into your own leadership style. Keep in mind that no matter what style you choose for yourself, authenticity is of the utmost importance in creating a sense of trust and confidence in your followers.

Directive leaders make decisions on their own and define clear roles and expectations for follower performance. Participative leaders let followers make decisions as the team or organization progresses toward goal attainment. Transformational leaders inspire confidence in their followers. They charismatically articulate a vision and lift their followers to achieve feats far greater than they may think possible. A leader who incorporates into his or her mission the development and empowerment of his or her followers is displaying a servant leadership style. In this approach to leadership, the organization is believed to be only as good as the followers whom the leader helps develop. Thus, the servant leader does everything in his or her power to make sure his or her followers succeed.

**Leading Change**
Organizational change is hard. Many organizations have institutionalized systems of accountability and sustainability linked to specific ways of accomplishing tasks. People become stuck in their ways because the systems in which they operate facilitate normative behavior—behavior regulated by tradition and expectation instead of behavior enlivened by innovation and aspiration. As we have previously stated, the profession of pharmacy has relied heavily on leaders acting as change agents to advance practice standards. Understanding tactics successfully used by organizations in creating change is a critical first step toward becoming a change agent.

Kotter has studied hundreds of organizations with a keen interest on understanding how leaders act as change agents within their organization (Reference 5). Through his research, he identified eight steps that leaders should perform to be successful change agents: create a sense of urgency necessitating change, build a powerful group to oversee the change, create a vision, communicate the vision, empower others to action, create and reward incremental changes, create organizational change, and develop organizational systems to permanently sustain changes. Embed these eight steps into your leadership tool kit, and practice as many of these actions as you possibly can. You may not encounter an opportunity to facilitate an entire organizational change during your time as a student because successful organizational change may take several years. However, by practicing and honing your skills in these areas, you will be empowered and able to be that change agent your practice site and the profession need when the time comes.

## MANAGEMENT

B.D. is a 20-year-old Pharm.D. student in his first professional year at the University of Iowa. He has many ambitions: good grades, an active social life, and a residency after pharmacy school. After 1 week of classes, B.D. seems distraught with the vast amount of material he needs to learn and begins to second-guess his ability to accomplish his goals. He wants to find ways to succeed in pharmacy school. What can B.D. do to better manage himself and others in accomplishing his goals? How can management help him be a distinguishable resident candidate?

All too often, the terms *leadership* and *management* are used interchangeably. They most certainly should not be, however, and those who do so fail to comprehend the underlying premises that differentiate each term. Although good leaders must be good managers, not all good managers are good leaders (Reference 6). In the sections that follow, we provide some salient thoughts on what it takes to become a good manager. And, once again, your personal success as a manager will likely come through a series of incremental steps that, collectively and over time, will help you acquire and refine your managerial skills.

### Management Functions and Levels

The activities performed by a manager can be grouped into four broad management functions: plan, organize, direct, and evaluate (Reference 7). A manager is required to make many decisions when managing complex organizations. Managers must consider both the long- and short-term implications of actions they are considering as well as the many resources, both human and capital, involved in carrying out those actions. In addition, they should consider how the timing of their actions affects the course their plan will follow. These deliberations, conducted either alone or with a team, are considered planning. Once decisions have been made, managers are responsible for organizing. People, materials, and other resources need to be arranged to maximize efficiency. Managers will then direct the allocation of organized resources so that, as tasks are completed, they can evaluate performance and analyze outcomes. These analyses can be used for subsequent decisions, should additional work need to be accomplished.

These management functions are used by managers in a variety of levels (Reference 7). The first level of management is self-management. Leaders and managers need to manage themselves before they can manage others. Being able to manage your time is a big component of self-management, especially during pharmacy school. Managers responsible for more than just themselves are working as interpersonal leaders. These leaders are found in the community and other volunteer organizations. Managers also operate in organizations starting at the team level. These mid-managers are responsible for a group of individuals within a larger organization. For example, the director of an inpatient pharmacy service in a health system is a team manager. Finally, organizational managers can be system-wide managers. These are the executive or board level managers of the organization responsible for the entire operation. Because being a good self-manager is necessary for engaging in management functions at higher levels, we will address self-management first.

Developing skills in time and project management can help you fulfill the obligations of both student and leader roles. Time management skills can help you prioritize tasks, exert personal effort in a coordinated manner, and reflect on successes and shortcomings in achieving your desired goals. Project management skills can be used alone or in conjunction with a team to help define project objectives, complete tasks in a timely manner, evaluate performance, and finalize the project. Both of these skills draw heavily on the management functions of plan-organize-direct-evaluate. Table 1 presents an overview of available time and project management actions or strategies. These strategies are also discussed in the following sections.

## Time Management

As a pharmacy student, you will have many competing demands for your time. With all the rigors of the classroom, many experiential practice experiences, and boundless professional opportunities, it may be difficult

**Table 1.** Strategies and Tactics of Time and Project Management

| Management Functions | Time Management | Project Management |
|---|---|---|
| Plan | SMART goals | Goals/objectives/action plans |
| Organize | Covey's four quadrants<br>Prioritization | Resource acquisition<br>Performance metrics |
| Direct | Scheduling<br>Taking action | Meetings<br>Delegation |
| Evaluate | Reflection | Project evaluation |

SMART = specific, reasonable, assignable, realistic, and time-related.

to have time for a personal life. Although many people desire to achieve a work-life balance, this philosophic approach to time management may be unobtainable for most pharmacy students. A more methodical approach to time management is through a process of prioritization, taking action, and engaging in purposeful reflection that will allow you to control the effort exerted on the activities you choose to fulfill both your personal and professional goals.

*Setting SMART Goals*

By establishing your goals in a formalized manner, you can avoid the many pitfalls people face in time management. Thus, you should begin your quest in time management by thinking about what you want to accomplish. The acronym SMART stands for a strategy you can use to help establish goals. Goals are smart if they are specific, reasonable, assignable, realistic, and time-related (Reference 8). A common goal of pharmacy students is to "become more involved." Although being involved is very important, it is difficult to accomplish if thought of in such a vague way. Applying the SMART principles will increase the likelihood of this goal being accomplished.

What specifically do you want to be involved in? Do you have a favorite student organization? Does your college offer opportunities for students to volunteer at public events or on committees? By defining specifically what you want to be involved in, you can begin planning other aspects necessary to attain the goal. Being able to precisely measure goal processes and outcomes is the next criteria. How many meetings will you attend? How many events will you participate in? Setting your involvement expectations in a quantifiable way will allow you to determine your success in attaining the goal. In our involvement example, the goal is yours alone. However, not every goal will only involve you, and soliciting the help of others may be necessary. Thus, assigning specific portions of the goal to others should be done next.

After you determine the specifics, measures, and assignments for the goal, spend time evaluating how realistic it is. In our involvement example, you could ask yourself, "Can I commit to one organization, three meetings, and one public service event?" Finally, place a timeframe on completing the goal. Our involvement example can likely be completed in a single semester. So the involvement goal went from "being more involved" to "participating in one professional organization by attending three meetings and helping with one public service event during the next semester." This goal has a greater likelihood of being completed, and even if it is not, you will be able to determine where and why your effort came up short. (See also Step I: Define (and Redefine) Your Goals for more guidance on goal setting.)

### Prioritization and Covey's Time Management Matrix

Prioritization should occur long before things happen. You already committed to prioritization when you decided to spend time reading this book. You are interested in pursuing a residency and have begun thinking about what needs to be done and when it should occur. This type of long-term thinking is critical to meeting the goal of obtaining a residency position. But do not limit yourself there. Prioritization is useful for all goals. Begin thinking about personal accomplishments or objectives you would like to complete in the next 2–5 years. Then begin thinking about all the steps that could help you achieve these goals. By prioritizing both professional and personal long-term goals now, you will build a strong foundation for planning your efforts during pharmacy school.

One way of thinking about how to allocate and organize the limited amount of time you have available is to use Covey's time management matrix (Reference 9). Covey suggests that every activity a person spends time performing can be categorized using two criteria, importance and urgency. That means that activities can fall into one of four quadrants: activities with high importance and high urgency, activities with high importance and low urgency, activities with low importance and high urgency, and activities with low importance and low urgency.

Quadrant 1 activities are those that are both important and urgent. Deadlines and unplanned projects or crises fit into this category. Quadrant 2 activities are those that are important, but not urgent. Developing relationships with colleagues and participating in professional association events are examples from pharmacy school. Also, planned projects and scheduled exams fit into this category, assuming you put in enough preparation to prevent them from being urgent. Quadrant 3 activities are those that are not important, but urgent. These are often certain phone calls, e-mails, and other interruptions that people deal with throughout the day. Quadrant 4 activities are those that are not urgent and not important. These can include browsing the Internet and other unfocused time wasters.

By focusing most of your efforts on activities that fit into quadrant 2, you can have less stress, experience more satisfaction, and achieve higher levels of motivation necessary to accomplish long-term goals (Reference 9). Covey's time management matrix provides one strategy to use in deciding how to allocate your time, with a focus on maximizing your success in achieving long-term goals.

*Scheduling, Taking Action, and Reflection*
Several tools can assist you in scheduling the tasks you want to accomplish. Although it is not important to discuss them all here, it is important for you to choose and use the scheduling tool that works best for you. By scheduling tasks in a systematic way using a calendar or other planning tool, you can commit yourself to completing that activity in a given amount of time. This does not mean that if you go over the time allotted, you must panic. That happens. What it does mean is that you will be empowered to look back on what you accomplished and failed to accomplish with a way to identify how you allocated and used time to complete tasks.

Reflection is a powerful, metacognitive process that humans have the ability to perform. How do you know when you did something well or not? Instead of waiting for someone else to answer that question for you, self-starters will ask themselves if they accomplished everything they desired. By asking yourself reflective questions, you have assumed responsibility and have begun to explore how your actions influenced the outcomes achieved, both good and bad. This process provides you with information necessary to achieve more efficient results the next time you act. We all know there are times in our lives when certain obligations will outweigh others—an important exam is coming up, or residency applications are coming due. Sacrifices will be made in such a way that a balance is highly unlikely. By engaging in reflection, you can align and realign your time management goals and act accordingly.

## Project Management

Throughout your personal and professional life, you will want to accomplish goals and objectives related to a particular project. Project management is a form of interpersonal management used to complete projects as a team by using the tenets of management. These tenets can help you break down your project into manageable components, provide direction to others through delegating authority, and evaluate the performance related to completing project goals. Your projects can be completed to the highest standard of excellence, and you will hone your management skills by taking a managerial approach to completing projects while in pharmacy school.

### *Creating Goals, Objectives, Action Plans, and Performance Metrics*

The first step to developing a successful project is to think about what you want to accomplish. As mentioned earlier, the SMART strategy may be useful in this process. However, in project management, the issue of measurability is of increased importance because of the many tasks that need to be completed simultaneously and the vast resources involved in many projects. Thus, expanding your initial goal planning to include the development of objectives and action plans is important. Objectives can be considered smaller units of goals. These smaller units typically involve a single aspect of a project goal. For example, say your project goal is to develop a community service project to screen patients for hypertension within the semester. Objectives for this type of goal could include developing hypertension screening competencies of pharmacy students, developing relationships with a screening site, and developing relationships with faculty and other pharmacists having an interest in cardiovascular disease management. By breaking a goal into smaller objectives, you have developed a framework for the actions needed to fulfill your goal.

Action plans are specific tasks assigned to one person that can be completed by a certain date. More people can help complete these action steps, but one person must be given responsibility for ensuring the task is done at the scheduled time. Action plans for developing pharmacy student competencies could be to schedule a training session, secure faculty involvement, and market a training session to targeted students. When these tasks are done, a training session will occur, and the pharmacy student's competencies should increase. These increased competencies, the expected outcome, can be measured and analyzed so you can know whether your project was successful.

Developing specific action plans or tactics for completing each goal and objective can serve as the basis for developing performance metrics, or indicators of successful completion of a project. An electronic or paper-based spreadsheet is useful when developing a set of performance metrics. Goals, objectives, and action plans are placed in the spreadsheet. In another column, you can list the time for completing each action plan. In addition, outputs, or products of action, should be placed in another column. Finally, a person is assigned to complete each action plan, and his or her name is placed in another column. For example, if one action plan is to contact faculty interested in teaching pharmacy students about hypertension screening, a column would be created for the anticipated deadline, and another column would be created to note that an e-mail communication would be sent and by whom. As action plans are worked on, a marking system can be used to indicate completeness. Table 2 provides a sample of a goal, objective, and action plans mapped out on a spreadsheet.

One thing to consider when developing action plans and performance metrics for your project is the depth of management you will provide. That is, you must decide how small or detailed the objectives and action plans will be for each project goal. Although outlining as many actions as possible to complete a project may intuitively seem useful, it may indeed be counterproductive. Ideally, your action plans should be specific enough to achieve a minimum standard. However, they need not be so specific that they are perceived of as micromanaging. This style of management can stifle creativity and minimize motivation for people assisting in project completion. Find a balance between control and flexibility when creating action plans to avoid these pitfalls.

*Meetings and Delegation*
In directing aspects of the project, meetings and delegation are two important tactics a manager may use. Meetings are structured gatherings of selected members of a team. They may be open to all members of the team or only to certain members, depending on the topics being discussed. Meetings work best when a clear agenda is set with input from all participants. An agenda outlines the topics for discussion, any action that is expected to take place at the meeting, and the suggested amount of time dedicated to each topic. E-mailing the agenda a day or two ahead of time gives meeting participants a chance to prepare for the discussion. When conducting the meeting, it is important to start and end on time as a way to show your respect for meeting participants (Reference 10). Meetings work most effectively when there are ground

**Table 2.** Sample Goal, Objective, and Action Plan Spreadsheet

| Goal(s) | Objective(s) | Action Plan(s) | Person(s) Responsible | Date to Be Completed | Completed |
|---|---|---|---|---|---|
| I. To provide a free medical clinic service to the community | A. Market free medical clinic services to community | 1. Create flyers. | BJP | 1/30/13 | |
| | | 2. Create newspaper advertisement. | DEL | 1/23/13 | |
| | | | | | |
| | | | | | |

rules dictating appropriate behavior for meeting participants. Although it is unnecessary for all meetings to be run according to the strict *Robert's Rules of Order*, having a principle of one person speaking at a time and allowing each person to speak on a topic once before people are allowed to speak again could be useful. Meetings are an important means of facilitating two-way communication toward attaining project goals. Judicious use of meetings for important decisions can facilitate team performance.

Delegation is the act of a manager giving authority to a follower to complete a task for which the manager is ultimately responsible. Delegation works best when the task being delegated is narrowly defined, the follower is capable of completing the task, and the manager instills confidence and trust in the follower completing the task (Reference 11). Tasks being delegated should not be meaningless, nor should they be something the manager has sole authority for doing. For example, it would not be appropriate to delegate conducting performance reviews of pharmacy staff or doing the paperwork associated with performance reviews. However, it could be appropriate to delegate a process that gathers feedback for improving performance reviews and providing recommendations for changes. By delegating meaningful tasks, you will help followers develop personally and as members of the team.

*Project Evaluation*
Evaluating the outcomes achieved versus those desired is the critical component of project evaluation. In essence, were you successful? If you systematically developed and tracked performance metrics for each goal and objective, you did the hard work associated with project evaluation. If you did not track those data, you will need to gather similar information using another means. Having a meeting with other

**Table 3.** Recommended Leadership and Management Activities for the Pharmacy Student by Professional Year

| Professional Year | Recommended Leadership and Management Activities |
|---|---|
| P1 | • Build self-management and interpersonal management skills.<br>• Join a professional or civic organization.<br>• Find a mentor to help you develop leadership skills. |
| P2 | • Serve on committees in professional or civic organization.<br>• Take leadership coursework or attend leadership seminars.<br>• Serve in small leadership role. |
| P3 | • Serve on committees in professional or civic organization.<br>• Take leadership coursework or attend leadership seminars.<br>• Serve in larger leadership role. |
| P4 | • Participate in an administrative-focused rotation. |

key leaders and followers to debrief the outcomes of your efforts is important. You can share experiences that led to success or failure in achieving the desired goals and objectives. It also gives you a chance to formally reward the team's efforts in the presence of their peers and colleagues. Reflection on and introspection of the team's accomplishments can lead to more focused work on the next project.

## BECOMING A PHARMACY STUDENT LEADER (AND MANAGER)

Leadership and management skills are not intended to be used infrequently. Development and refinement of your skills will only come with use. Table 3 has suggestions for actions you can take throughout your pharmacy education to increase your leadership and management skills.

As reflected in this guide, a student can hone leadership and management skills in several ways. So, the question isn't availability; opportunities to lead and manage abound. Rather, the key question is whether you will choose to take advantage of the many opportunities that exist for you to become a good leader and manager. Is there a willingness to do so? Is there a burning desire to set yourself apart from others by making the difficult decisions and taking on projects or pursuing opportunities that others shy away from? That you are reading this guide suggests strongly that you have the motivation it takes to do so. Seeking leadership and management opportunities will help you lay the foundation needed to pursue challenging opportunities including residency training.

> *Holding a leadership position in pharmacy school allowed me not only to advance my own leadership skills, but also to contribute to the advancement of pharmacy practice. I am excited to be part of a profession that will consistently challenge me to move forward.*
>
> —Aimee Loucks, 2012/13 PGY2 Drug Information Specialty Resident at Kaiser Permanente, Oakland, Calif.

Take advantage of every opportunity to lead and manage. Each time you take on such a challenge, you arm yourself with more leadership and management skills than you had before. In doing so, you will feel a sense of pride and accomplishment by knowing that your community (academic, professional, or civic) is benefiting from your efforts … efforts that reflect your growth as a leader and manager.

As noted at the beginning of this chapter, residency program directors are looking for candidates with proven leadership and management potential. Residency program directors and others who precept residents know that, under their tutelage, building on students' leadership and management skills helps develop a new generation of change agents who can further advance the profession. So, go ahead, take advantage of opportunities to lead and manage. Pursue those challenges. What are you waiting for? The world needs change agents. The world needs you.

## REFERENCES

1. Avolio BJ. Leadership Development in Balance: MADE/Born. Mahwah, NJ: Lawrence Erlbaum Associates, 2005.
2. Lansing A. Endurance: Shackleton's Incredible Voyage. New York: Basic Books, 1999.
3. White SJ. Leadership: successful alchemy. Am J Health Syst Pharm 2006;63:1497-503.
4. Boleman LG, Deal TE. Reframing Organizations. San Francisco: Jossey-Bass, 2008.
5. Kotter JP. Leading change: why transformation efforts fail. Harv Bus Rev 1995;Mar/Apr:59-67.
6. Fabricators and Manufacturers of America. 2003. Managers Are Not Necessarily Leaders. Available at www.thefabricator.com/article/forceos/managers-are-not-necessarily-leaders. Accessed September 13, 2012.
7. Zgarrick DP. Management functions. In: Deselle SP, Zgarrick DP, Alston GL, eds. Pharmacy Management, 3rd ed. New York: McGraw-Hill, 2012.
8. Doran GT. There's a SMART way to write management's goals and objectives. Manag Rev 1981;70:35-6.
9. Covey SR. The 7 Habits of Highly Effective People. New York: Simon and Schuster, 1989.
10. Saenz R, Mark SM, Vaillancourt AM. Managing your time. In: Chisholm-Burns MA, Vaillancourt AM, Shepherd M, eds. Pharmacy Management, Leadership, Marketing, and Finance. Sudbury, MA: Jones & Bartlett, 2011.
11. Mark SM, Saenz R. Management essentials for pharmacists. In: Chisholm-Burns MA, Vaillancourt AM, Shepherd M. Pharmacy Management, Leadership, Marketing, and Finance. Sudbury, MA: Jones & Bartlett, 2011.

# STEP V
# GAIN VALUABLE WORK EXPERIENCE

Stephen F. Eckel, Pharm.D., MHA, BCPS

## ABBREVIATIONS IN THIS CHAPTER

ACPE     Accreditation Council for Pharmacy Education
APPE     Advanced pharmacy practice experience
IPPE      Introductory pharmacy practice experience
RPD      Residency program director

## INTRODUCTION

Many pharmacy students originally become interested in this profession through their experience working at a local pharmacy. Although some may have held positions as pharmacy technicians, many others were able to see the benefits of pharmacy through observing and talking to pharmacists about aspects of their job, including the satisfaction associated with it. In addition to the ways in which work experience helps people make career choices, pharmacy schools recognize the benefits of work experience as a potential factor in the admissions process (Reference 1).

    As students pursue their pharmacy degree, many continue to work weekends and summers in their original workplace. Others recognize the importance of getting a pharmacy-related job while in school, either to help them in their classes or to pay the rising cost of tuition and the many expenses associated with being a student. One study found that almost 100% of all students surveyed had a job by the time they reached their advanced pharmacy practice experiences (APPEs), with more than 75% of them employed in a community pharmacy (Reference 2).

Some pharmacists who graduated years ago had to document so many hours of work experience (internship) before becoming eligible for licensure. This was usually 1,500 hours, which was required for pharmacists to be eligible to take the state license exam. Although some states still have this requirement, many others allow the APPEs mandated by the Accreditation Council for Pharmacy Education (ACPE) to count for all the required work hours needed to take the state license exam. Thus, it is possible that a pharmacy student entering a residency program has limited-to-no consistent work experience in a pharmacy. This raises many questions; for instance, is this approach less than optimal, as viewed by those involved in residency candidate selection? What are the benefits and concerns to the residency candidate of pharmacy-related work experience? Does it matter what type of employment the pharmacy student engages in? Although these types of questions have no definite answers and opinions will surely differ, this chapter will describe the potential benefits or downsides of employment and reasons that appropriate pharmacy work experience may assist students in improving their opportunities to secure a residency position.

## GAINING WORK EXPERIENCE IN YOUR CURRICULUM

Each graduate of an ACPE-accredited school of pharmacy is required to complete an introductory pharmacy practice experience (IPPE). This encompasses 2 months of overview experiences, strategically placed early in the curriculum. Each pharmacy student has 1 month in community pharmacy and 1 month in hospital pharmacy. The student is also required to complete no less than 1,440 hours (36 weeks) of APPEs during the final academic year (Reference 3). The structure of APPEs is left up to the academic institution to decide, but most experiences need to be in the following settings: community pharmacy, hospital or health system pharmacy, ambulatory care, and inpatient/acute care general medicine (Reference 3). The sum of these experiences equates to about 9 months of training during the final year or, applying this to the working world, three summers of internships. Each school of pharmacy has its own nuances on how APPE rotations need to be configured. Some colleges require more community pharmacy–based experiences, whereas others expect more experiences in the acute care or hospital setting. Some schools of pharmacy are affiliated with an academic medical center, allowing students to complete many of their hospital rotations there. At schools not located near a hospital or not closely affiliated with an academic medical center, students might try to independently find APPE rotations that provide better preparation for residency training than the ones currently offered. Even though there are requirements regarding what pharmacy students need to do during their experiential education experience, tremendous variability exists in their training among students at various programs, even within the same school of pharmacy. Because of this, it is important to find additional avenues to experience and learn about a pharmacist's daily activities.

Although pharmacy students are not compensated for participating in experiential training, some aspects of both choosing and completing APPE experiences may contribute to becoming a stronger residency candidate. These include the engagement of students on APPE rotations. Some pharmacy students are active members of the patient care team or pharmacy, whereas others take the role of an observer. Students may choose to passively watch what is occurring in the medical decision-making process for the patient, but if so, they should never have the expectation of being responsible for the actual decision or even of attending rounds for hospital-based rotations. Pharmacy students should strive to maximize their participation and get the most from their APPEs because this will be the foundation for success in the residency interview process and subsequently in being a resident. With the type of variability in rotations that exists and the recognition of what a residency requires from an individual, most residency program directors (RPDs) understand that the APPEs all pharmacy students experience do not fully prepare them for the role of a pharmacy resident. Even though a state board of pharmacy might count the 1,440 hours of experiential education as enough "work experience" to qualify for licensure, the variability of experiences, the activities the student completed on rotation, the differences in rotation required, and the type of institution in which students practiced do not fully prepare students for excelling in a residency program. However, there are ways to maximize the opportunities that exist (see Step VI: Maximize Experiential Education).

The IPPEs can provide an excellent overview about different career tracks. You will have the opportunity to observe various practice sites to see which one appeals to you. If one is found to be advantageous, you can make decisions to get more and varied exposure to this setting. In addition, it could lead to future employment opportunities, both as you gain experiences with a site and as the pharmacy learns about you.

The APPEs are structured to give you more in-depth experiences in the various practice settings. If you select the APPEs such that your clinical rotations are completed before the residency showcase at the American Society of Health-System Pharmacists Midyear Clinical Meeting in December, your passion for this practice setting and daily activities could lead you to pursue a residency. In addition, strong clinical experiences in either the acute or ambulatory care setting could be viewed as good preparation for a residency and something to share when talking about previous experiences. Unfortunately, not everyone can have success in aligning rotations and sites perfectly, so do not get frustrated if this happens. The APPEs are only one aspect of the spectrum of work experiences described in this chapter.

## VARIETY OF WORK EXPERIENCE

There are different work environments in which you might choose to seek employment. Most students, however, will work in the community pharmacy setting. The positions are plentiful, the hours are typically more flexible than in a hospital setting, and you can often work across different stores within the same chain. In addition, many other students have worked in this environment before enrolling in pharmacy school. A smaller percentage of students work in the hospital setting. These jobs are typically more difficult to get, especially if the hospital is located in the same area as the school of pharmacy. This is because fewer of these opportunities exist. These positions can be more limited regarding flexibility with the schedule and usually require you to work during holidays and throughout the summer. Finally, you may choose to work in nontraditional areas. These include the pharmaceutical industry, home infusion companies, and nuclear pharmacy, to name a few. If you have community pharmacy experience before entering pharmacy school, you may choose to broaden your experience by seeking employment in one of these different areas. You could also choose jobs that have nothing to do with pharmacy at all but that strengthen other important skills. For example, tutoring chemistry students can advance your teaching skills, and leading campus tours can improve your public speaking abilities.

Another possibility is taking advantage of summer internships. Not only are these usually time-limited (i.e., one summer), but they also provide experiences to work in different parts of the country and enable you to see the variability in pharmacy practice. These are also very competitive, so it is important to distinguish your application from those of others. Internship opportunities exist in the federal government, pharmaceutical industry, community pharmacy corporate offices, and academic medical centers, for example. These are wonderful experiences through which to learn and broaden your network.

If you have recognized that the sector of pharmacy of interest to you is not the one in which you are currently working, there are ways to get exposure to those settings other than the workplace. Reaching out to a pharmacist to ask about volunteering or shadowing can create a better appreciation of what other settings are like. This can be accomplished through several different avenues. Contacting a faculty member with an active practice, asking faculty for different names at a specific institution, reaching out to pharmacists from your hometown, or asking a resident or a student on rotation are all good ways to contact appropriate people for shadowing experiences. Experiences that can occur during these times include attending rounds, talking about the positive and negative aspects of the job, reviewing patient profiles, conducting a patient workup, or counseling a patient. Unfortunately, it is sometimes difficult to get shadowing opportunities with a pharmacist because of the busyness of his or her schedule. Being patient and working around the pharmacist's schedule is sometimes necessary to gain this exposure.

> One of the best things I did was search for a new job halfway through school. While I gained valuable experience as a community pharmacy intern, I knew I was interested in pursuing residency and thus wanted to work in the hospital setting. I was worried that no one would want to hire me since they would only get to keep me for less than two years prior to graduation, but I tried anyway. Getting hired as a hospital pharmacy intern provided me with many valuable skills and knowledge that I still use today as a PGY2 resident.
>
> —Deborah Raithel, 2012/13 PGY2 Pediatrics Resident at University of Illinois at Chicago, Chicago, Ill.

Local hospitals usually have volunteer offices, and if they know you are a pharmacy student, they can usually prioritize your time to the pharmacy department. Although some of the activities that can be done are menial, the networking and observational exposures can potentially open up future opportunities. Another fantastic opportunity is participating in a service-learning project. These are usually free clinics offered in many locations, and they are frequently looking for assistance with the pharmacy. This could include providing immunizations, taking medication histories, conducting a medication review, determining what available products could treat a specific condition, or educating patients about their medications.

Although such activities do not replace employment in these settings, you can get a feel for the "typical" day of a pharmacist. These opportunities can be used to confirm your interests, guide future experiential education placement, or create opportunities to get involved in projects or other learning experiences.

Schools of pharmacy can also provide unique experiences if you are interested in pursuing a residency. Many students can work as teaching assistants or even have the opportunity to lecture in a class or gain experience working in a lab with research-based faculty. Schools of pharmacy may also offer an academic rotation, which could be good exposure to academia and teaching. This is a great career opportunity, but few students gain exposure to it. Many times, you will need to seek out the opportunities because they may not be readily apparent. Given that residency requirements often include education and conducting a project, RPDs often view research involvement, publications, and classroom teaching as favorable activities. These types of experiences are good to share on a residency interview and may lead to further opportunities for diversifying your experiences.

Employment opportunities can be found through talking with faculty, residents, and other students. In addition, schools of pharmacy or universities will have career development offices, where there is access to internships and other opportunities. Reaching out to leaders in professional associations or just searching the Internet is an avenue you can use to find opportunities for employment or internship experiences.

Although there is no "right" place for you to work when you wish to maximize your chances of getting a residency position, it is important to fully optimize the benefits of the work experience. This includes taking advantage of the opportunities presented, developing relationships with people employed there, and making a good impression with a positive work ethic.

## BENEFITS OF WORK EXPERIENCE

The potential benefits of having a job during pharmacy school are many, some of which are listed in Box 1. In addition, the experiences and advantages of employment can lead you to be more competitive and prepared for the interview and subsequent residency training.

When you work in a pharmacy during school, you are exposed to certain tasks that often match nicely with what is taught in the classroom setting. You are required to learn brand and generic names; how to communicate, both verbally and nonverbally, with patients and health care providers; and how to become competent in the basics of compounding and aseptic technique, to name a few topics. These are all activities performed by pharmacists on a daily basis that offer great exposure and learning opportunities. Because these tasks are taught and subsequently tested, you are in a position to enhance your performance in the classroom setting. Even though prior work experience has not been correlated to better academic or clinical performance, it can still increase your confidence and awareness (Reference 4). In addition, you may learn new skills through the classroom setting that you can bring back to the workplace to help improve your delivery of patient care. Although residency programs don't just focus on grades, excelling in the classroom setting will make your application that much more competitive.

A second benefit of working when you are a pharmacy student is gaining a better understanding of what a pharmacist does. There are positive and negative aspects to any job, and working in different practice settings can allow you to be exposed to them. You can also observe what skills are necessary for this work setting and determine whether the environment is a good match as a career path. In the hospital setting, you will be exposed to several different roles, even those you may not participate in directly. Besides the central pharmacy and IV room, where most students work, there are clinical pharmacy activities and administrative responsibilities that might appeal to you. Even if you have no desire for full-time employment where you currently work, this experience will provide valuable information. Employment in a pharmacy-related position may provide career guidance and insight on

---

**Box 1.** Tangible benefits of work experience during pharmacy school.

- Potential for improved performance in the classroom setting
- Better understanding of the responsibilities of a pharmacist
- Career assessment and planning
- Networking with pharmacists and other health care providers
- Potential of better preparation for APPEs (advanced pharmacy practice experiences)
- Development of time management skills
- Development of professionalism
- Licensure-ready for states still requiring work experience
- Previous interviewing experience for any position will provide practice for the all-important residency interview.

the next steps for the type of job to pursue. In addition, this experience leads to better assimilation into your residency training site. Not having to learn a new environment when starting a residency program will only bring early opportunities to experience different things and start your preparation for further training or employment.

Another positive outcome of working during pharmacy school is the relationships you develop through the workplace. The pharmacists will generally provide teaching and training opportunities for further learning if you have expressed this interest. Whether this is counseling a patient on a medication, eliciting a medication history, calculating a recommended dose according to the patient's pharmacokinetic parameters, or something else, there are great learning activities to be had. Other experiences you could have include involvement in a research study, coauthorship of a publication, or other activities typically not completed by a pharmacy student. Not only will you meet many pharmacists, but you will also get to know physicians, nurses, and patients. You will also better understand how pharmacy fits into the overall health care system. In addition, these relationships could create opportunities for you to get a positive letter of recommendation, which is a vital part of your residency application. Receiving a letter of recommendation from someone who knows you well is viewed positively by an RPD, especially if it is from a patient or nonpharmacist. Many times, this can only occur through relationships that evolve from the work setting.

In addition to being better prepared for the classroom setting, you may excel in the APPEs conducted in your work environment. Although being employed in a chain drug store does not mean you understand how an independent pharmacy operates, there are probably more similarities than differences. Thus, when you perform an APPE rotation in an independent pharmacy, you may not need to be taught fundamental tasks, such as how to dispense various medications, because you should already have adequate experience doing this. You can use this familiarity to become exposed to different and unique learning experiences compared with those not having this type of employment. If you have worked in the hospital setting, you should have a rudimentary appreciation of the medication use process. Although the technology and processes employed in each hospital are different, the fundamentals of how the medication reaches the patient are similar. If you have worked in the hospital setting, you may already have experience communicating with nurses and physicians on a frequent basis, so typically, you will not be as intimidated by this. You may also be able to better explain issues that arise because of the complexity in making or delivering an

IV that is hard to get in solution. Having this baseline experience will allow you to get beyond your introduction to the work setting and on to better learning opportunities.

One major item that all pharmacy residents face is how to manage so many competing activities. Residents need to know how to allocate time for an activity and how to limit procrastination. Students who have had jobs during pharmacy school understand this conundrum. Having an upcoming test on the same weekend as you have to work requires planning if you want to be successful in all activities. Your ability to handle competing demands during pharmacy school will show the RPD that you have modest time management skills and could successfully handle the demands of his or her residency. This should be balanced, however, with your individual academic performance; the quantity of work you do should not detract from course-related expectations, given that RPDs often consider GPAs part of the admissions process.

All students should strive toward professionalism in the work setting. Traits of a professional include a commitment to improve both knowledge and skills, conscientiousness, accountability for decisions, and the use of ethics in all settings (Reference 5). It is important that all residency candidates have a sense of professionalism, but this is a difficult trait to assess through the interview process. However, it has been determined that pharmacy work experience as a student, through observing the pharmacist, provides the beginnings of developing the traits of a professional (Reference 6). Thus, the workplace may serve as a venue for both the development and fostering of professional behavior, which should carry through to residency training.

As mentioned earlier, some states still require you to obtain internship hours to be eligible for state licensure. This is not a requirement in all states, however. If you attend school in a state where no such requirements exist, the student may not consider pharmacy employment because they do not see the potential benefit after reviewing other opportunities. However, when looking for residency positions, you will have to exclude yourself from applying to programs in states where the requirement for internship hours exists because you will be unable to get licensed as a pharmacist and complete the requirements for the residency program. Although no comprehensive list is known that gives the states and whether they require work hours for licensure, it is extremely important that you ask this question of the programs where you are unfamiliar with the state licensure expectations.

There are some potential downsides to employment. If you focus too much on employment, your grades could suffer because you have limited time to study. In addition, you might not have the opportunity to get as involved in professional student societies or to take valuable leadership positions. Also, an employer who is asked to write a letter of recommendation might have limited experience in writing these. You might also get excessively jaded perspectives about the profession, depending on the person you work with. This could be extremely deflating to you regarding the potential opportunities that exist with pharmacy. All of these could detract from your career direction and residency application. However, with careful planning from the beginning, employment could create opportunities to distinguish your portfolio of activities from those of other candidates.

Work experience may better prepare the student for a residency. Residency positions are becoming more competitive each year (Reference 7). The number of applications is growing beyond the number of positions being created. Thus, a prospective applicant needs to find ways to be distinguished from his or her peers. One method for this is to have pharmacy work experience. However, the experience itself is not what's important. It is how the applicant uses the employment to prepare for his or her future. This can be communicated through the cover letter, the answers to the essay questions (if applicable), the CV, and the letters of recommendation. The experiences and opportunities you gain can permeate all aspects of both your residency application and the interview. The RPD will be evaluating each candidate on how successful he or she will be in the program, and those who can communicate the value of their work experience will position themselves to be viewed favorably.

## INTERVIEW EXPERIENCE

When applying for jobs, one typically goes through an interview for the position. This experience is helpful when applying for a residency because all residency positions require an on-site interview. One of the techniques used for candidate selection today is called behavioral-based interviewing (Reference 8). As opposed to traditional interview-type questions, like "tell me why you are interested in this position" or "what would you do in this hypothetical situation," behavioral-based interviewing attempts to better understand the applicant's previous experiences and apply them to this position. A sample question is, "Tell me about a time that you had a difficult choice in front of you and how you specifically handled it." Other potential questions are found in Box 2. People who score higher on behavioral-based interviews can be a better fit for the position and more satisfied with the job, and they tend to stay in it longer. Residency programs are starting to use these questions as part of the interview process because they want the best fits and those with similar experiences for their residency program. Residency candidates who do better in these types of interviews are those with previous employment to draw on. The work setting is a good place to have specific, concrete examples that can be used to answer behavioral-based interview questions. Thus, you as a residency candidate who have had work experience may be in a better position to answer these questions, and if you answer them well, you will shine throughout the interview process. Even if the residency program does not use behavioral-based interviewing, practicing in advance is critical for success in an interview. Whether you use fellow students, faculty members, local residents, or pharmacists, going through mock interviews will give you an understanding of various questions that can be asked and a chance to practice answering them. It will also calm your nerves, knowing you have done this before and can confidently answer the questions that are asked.

## ADVICE TO THE RESIDENCY CANDIDATE
### Selecting a Job

If you are considering employment during pharmacy school and are not sure where to seek it, Box 3 has a few questions you may want to ask yourself. Although it is preferential to have work experience in the sector of pharmacy in which you want to pursue a residency, this is by no means required. Plenty of people have worked in the community

---

**Box 2.** Sample behavioral-based questions a pharmacy student could be asked.

- Tell me about a time when you dealt with an angry customer and how you handled the situation. What was the outcome?
- Give an example of how you have worked on a team.
- Describe a situation in which a member of a team you were on was not doing his or her part to make the rest of the team successful. What did you do to address the situation?
- Can you tell us about a time you went above and beyond to help a customer, patient, or coworker?
- Give an example of how you set goals and achieve them.
- Have you ever been in a situation where you didn't have enough work to do? If so, how did you handle it?

> **Box 3.** Questions to ask before seeking employment during pharmacy school.
>
> - Do I know which type of residency (community or hospital) I want to pursue? If so, it is preferential to work in this type of setting.
> - Will the time spent working significantly detract from my school-related responsibilities and potentially affect my grades?
> - Does the job require me to work summers and/or holidays?
> - Have I talked to others who had this position before? If so, were they generally positive regarding their experience?
> - What opportunities for continued growth exist with this position?
> - Have previous students with this job been successful in obtaining a residency position after they graduate?
> - Will work hours also count toward internship hours, if applicable?
> - Will taking this position minimize my involvement in other professional activities? If so, employment needs to be considered carefully.

pharmacy setting and have gone on to successfully complete pharmacy residencies. However, having hospital work experience and being able to communicate the benefits of this and specific activities that you performed on that job provide an opportunity to distinguish your skills from those of others. The most important issue is what you make of the experience. For example, two different pharmacy students work in the same community pharmacy. One comes to work dutifully each shift and does what is needed to get the job done. The other does not only the required activities, but also regularly asks the pharmacist questions that he or she does not know and asks for experience to do medication therapy management and patient education when the pharmacy is slow. It is not difficult to determine who is getting more out of the employment and who is better prepared to share lessons learned and experiences gained during a residency interview. The job has to be more than a place where you collect a paycheck; it must be something that teaches you about the profession of pharmacy, provides a network of individuals, and creates opportunities beyond the classroom setting.

## Summary

Work experience can be a valuable asset to any student wanting to obtain a pharmacy residency. Besides the economic advantages a job provides, work experience offers you the opportunity to perform better in your classes, refine your preferred future sector of employment, network with pharmacists and other health care providers who can offer opportunities for growth, excel on APPE rotations, develop good time management skills and professionalism, and gain experiences on which to share during the residency interview. Having these positive outcomes from the work experience will also allow your residency application to be distinguished from those of others. However, these opportunities are made; they do not just happen. Foresight, intentionality, balance with school-related activities, and planning can deliver these to every student who manages work experiences well.

## REFERENCES

1. Kelsch MP, Friesner DL. Evaluation of an interview process for admission into a school of pharmacy. Am J Pharm Educ 2012;76:22.
2. Siracuse MV, Schondelmeyer SW, Hadsall RS, Schommer JC. Third year pharmacy students' work experience and attitudes and perceptions of the pharmacy profession. Am J Pharm Educ 2008;72:50.
3. Accreditation Council for Pharmacy Education. Accreditation Standards and Guidelines for the Professional Program in Pharmacy Leading to the Doctor of Pharmacy Degree. Available at www.acpe-accredit.org/pdf/FinalS2007Guidelines2.0.pdf. Accessed September 19, 2012.
4. Mar E, Barnett MJ, T-L Tang T, Sasaki-Hill D, Kuperberg JR, Knapp K. Impact of previous pharmacy work experience on pharmacy school academic performance. Am J Pharm Educ 2010;74:42.
5. White paper on pharmacy student professionalism. J Am Pharm Assoc (Wash) 2000;40:96-102.
6. Schafheutle EI, Hassell K, Ashcroft DM, et al. How do pharmacy students learn professionalism? Int J Pharm Pract 2012;20:118-28.
7. ASHP & Commission on Credentialing Updates. Available at www.ashp.org/DocLibrary/Accreditation/ASDMCMTownHall2011.aspx. Accessed September 19, 2012.
8. Quintessential Careers: Behavioral Job Interviewing Strategies for Job-Seekers: http://www.quintcareers.com/behavioral_interviewing.html. Accessed October 2, 2012.

# STEP VI

# MAXIMIZE EXPERIENTIAL EDUCATION

Brian L. Erstad, Pharm.D., FCCP, BCPS;
and Marcella Hoyland, Pharm.D., BCPS

## HOW MAXIMIZING EXPERIENTIAL ROTATIONS WILL HELP SECURE A RESIDENCY

Experiential education is your ticket to the world of pharmacy. You will meet many preceptors along the way in various clinical settings, from community practice to academia to clinical pharmacy and management positions, to name a few. The wide array of options is one of the reasons many students choose pharmacy as a profession. Although the choices can be overwhelming, the opportunities are immense, and you should take advantage of them.

You will be exposed to many different practice settings by the introductory pharmacy practice experiences (IPPEs) throughout your didactic years and the advanced pharmacy practice experiences (APPEs) in your fourth professional year. During these experiences, you will not only be exposed to a potential future career option, but also gain one-on-one time with your assigned preceptor. So put your best foot forward.

Doing well during your IPPEs and APPEs will allow you many avenues of opportunity. You want to be a standout student because your pharmacy practice experiences will often lead to mentors and letters of recommendation. Performing well during each of your experiences will make a lasting impression on your preceptors. Your preceptors and other pharmacists at your experiential sites can give you advice on career choices and help you make these choices a reality by writing and speaking of your value to the pharmacy community. You want to be true to yourself to help narrow your interests, which will perhaps lead to specialty areas you may pursue (e.g., ambulatory care, cardiology, critical care, infectious diseases, nuclear, nutrition, oncology, pediatrics, psychiatry). By asking questions and taking steps in each of your preceptor's shoes, experiential education can help guide the choices you make regarding residency—and ultimately, your career as a pharmacist. Finally, you want to do your best work to help develop the skills and knowledge necessary to secure a residency and become a successful pharmacy practice resident.

### INVESTING IN YOUR OWN EDUCATION

Congratulations, you are ready to embark on some of the most important training of your career, experiential education. It begins with your IPPEs. The Accreditation Council for Pharmacy Education suggests that students experience at least 300 IPPE hours during the first three professional years. Introductory pharmacy practice experiences are to be balanced between community and institutional settings for a minimum of 150 hours, allowing 20% of IPPEs (e.g., 60 hours of 300 hours) to be simulations, practical laboratories, objective structured clinical examinations, and so forth (Reference 1). Introductory pharmacy practice experiences have been developed to help the early pharmacy student apply knowledge from the classroom to patient care while under a preceptor's comfort and close supervision. Introductory pharmacy practice experiences are often intermingled within the curriculum, depending on the specific school or college of pharmacy you attend, and provide an opportunity to ask questions and clarify key concepts learned in the classroom. Take advantage of this situation. Do not grow frustrated when your questions are answered with questions; you will not be able to answer everything, nor are you expected to. Instead, impress your preceptor by coming to the experience well-read and willing to research the answers to the preceptor's questions. Be enthusiastic and ready to learn; this is your first impression on the pharmacy community.

Making a good impression and performing well during the IPPEs will only help, not hinder, you during your APPEs. Advanced pharmacy practice experiences will take place during your fourth professional year for at least 1440 hours (i.e., 36 weeks), with required rotations in community pharmacy, hospital or health-system pharmacy, ambulatory care, and inpatient/acute care general medicine, allowing the remaining hours to be dedicated to elected rotations geared toward your individual interests (Reference 1). Often, your APPEs will occur in the same institution as a previously completed IPPE and/or your IPPE and APPE preceptors will know each other; therefore, your reputation can speak volumes, both good and bad. Performing well is not only to your intellectual advantage, but also to your professional advantage in fostering relationships with the pharmacy community, creating a well-known reputation, and ultimately, securing a residency.

## PROFESSIONALISM

A section on professionalism might seem superfluous in this chapter, particularly because the traits of professionalism have been delineated for pharmacy practice (Reference 2), and surveys show that students recognize the importance of professionalism in pharmacy practice (References 3–5). However, many students are first exposed to interdisciplinary patient care activities during the IPPEs; moreover, this is when and where students interact with other health care professionals and begin to see their role as part of a health care team. Typically, this is also the student's first exposure to a pharmacist-preceptor and the level of professionalism upheld in the practice setting. Structured activities involving other health professions foster interdisciplinary understanding; so take advantage of such opportunities when available (Reference 6). Yet there is no substitute for learning the principles of professionalism through both your IPPEs and APPEs. These principles will foster interdisciplinary patient care through direct observation and modeling by experienced preceptors (References 7, 8).

A failed rotation could have career-altering consequences. One short-term consequence is the need for remediation, which could delay your graduation. Another likely consequence is the inability to obtain letters of recommendation from your rotation preceptors. If you are seeking postgraduate training or a clinical position, these letters are among the most important recommendations you will receive because they attest to your efforts in the clinical setting as opposed to the classroom. If remediation or unprofessional behavior occurs, the only reference of your clinical performance will be tarnished. From a longer-term perspective, always be cognizant that pharmacy is a small world, causing a suboptimal performance on an experiential rotation to have job implications beyond the immediate postgraduate period.

Of note, professionalism is a two-way street, meaning it is incumbent on your preceptor and other health professionals to model professional behaviors. Unfortunately, what is a professional or unprofessional behavior in the experiential setting is not always clear.

## Case Scenario

A male physician has not slept for more than 24 hours because of clinical responsibilities. You approach him with a suggestion for a change in therapy solely because of cost considerations, and he raises his voice to you in an insulting manner and refuses to take your suggestion. You have to ask yourself whether it is worth raising this issue at a higher administrative level through your preceptor or whether you should just write it off to a tired physician having a bad day. Additional context is very important for making this determination. If you have been interacting with this physician for some time and this is the first such episode, you may conclude it is an isolated event and not worthy of additional action other than mentioning the event to your preceptor. However, repetitive behavior by a physician that includes personal insults to you as a student is unprofessional and needs to be dealt with. In the latter situation, what you should not do is get into a verbal fight with the physician because this will accomplish nothing.

It is difficult to suggest one approach for handling such unprofessional verbal abuse, but in general, you should try to defuse and/or disengage from the situation and subsequently discuss the issue with your preceptor.

Hopefully, you will never again encounter such an extreme example of unprofessional behavior, but if you do, try not to let it make you cynical toward other health care professionals or extrapolate the behavior to a wide swath of physicians. Rather, set the example by showing you can rise above this type of altercation and continue to be collegial with other members of the health care team.

The preceding scenario discusses unprofessional behavior by another health care professional but does not address such behavior by other pharmacy students, pharmacist-residents, pharmacists, or even your immediate preceptor. For perceived unprofessional behavior by other pharmacy students, you could first try discussing your perception with the involved student in a calm, thoughtful manner. If this one-on-one conversation does not seem to work and the behavior seems to be repetitive, bring it up with your preceptor. When the behavior is by pharmacist-residents or other pharmacists, it is best to raise the issue directly with your preceptor. Not surprisingly, one of the more difficult situations is when you perceive unprofessional behavior by your preceptor toward you, your patients, or other health professionals. In the unlikely event this occurs, the context of the behavior (e.g., seriousness, repetitiveness) will help determine your action. For more serious and repetitive unprofessional behavior, you will need to raise the issue with the Office of Experiential Education (OEE). When bringing these situations to light with either your preceptor or the OEE, you must maintain your own professional composure. This is not the time to rant, rave, and point fingers; it is a time for a simple display of facts. Of importance, do not be accusatory in your conversation. Your goal should be to present the details of the situation; describe how it has affected you, the patient, the caregiver, the physician, and others; and ask for advice on how to help prevent future episodes.

## CRITICAL THINKING AND DEVELOPING A DEEPER UNDERSTANDING OF SUBJECT MATTER

Critical thinking generates learning beyond simple rote memorization (Reference 9). As a student, you are in essence taught to think with a skeptical mind but to remain empathetic toward the patient, all the while using a systematic approach to identifying and resolving potential or actual medication-related problems during your experiential training.

The first step is identifying the problem through data collection, gleaned from discussions with the patient or health care professionals, in conjunction with a thorough review of the patient's records. Second, propose potential solutions to the problem, and pick the solution that best optimizes benefits and reduces risks of harm for the individual patient.

Assuming your recommendation is implemented, test it to see if it works by controlling other factors as much as possible (e.g., limiting other concomitant changes that might obscure a proper assessment of the response) and by carefully monitoring the patient response. If your solution does not work—or works suboptimally—identify the best alternative solution and test it.

Even though these steps seem straightforward, the training needed to develop these skills at a higher level is not. Thus, the more years of experience through rotations as a student, followed by postgraduate training as a resident, the better your outcome.

## IPPE to APPE Progression

Other than sequence in the curriculum, the distinctions between IPPE and APPE rotations are not always clear-cut regarding student expectation. Because an APPE often occurs at the same site as a previously completed IPPE, you must be able to advance yourself and help the preceptor differentiate you from an IPPE student. For example, you will need more guidance in IPPE versus APPE rotations, and some IPPEs involve observational or modeled experiences; however, APPEs almost always involve direct patient care because there is no substitute for this type of hands-on training (Reference 10). Furthermore, as you progress through your IPPE and APPE rotations, you are expected to progress from simple abilities, such as knowledge and comprehension, to higher-order abilities, such as the ability to synthesize information and construct solutions to more complex patient care issues. Therefore, the difference in preceptor expectation between IPPEs and APPEs is tremendous.

Before the APPEs, your training involved abstract issues related to pharmacy practice and patient care. Now, it is time for the real thing. Ideally, at this point in your career development, you will grow to become a self-starter and self-learner, two qualities greatly desired by experiential preceptors. Sometimes, the didactic aspects of the pharmacy curriculum can foster unnecessary dependence on instructors by having everything set in stone with respect to class times, assignments, tests, and so forth. Thus, although you may have a comfort level in the classroom setting, things will start to change dramatically as you enter the APPE component of your curriculum. Suddenly, meetings and rounds may be at varying times because of the nature of the clinical arena. You will be expected to be prepared to research and discuss issues about which you may not have had in-depth didactic instruction. The instructor-student hierarchy in the classroom will change to an interdisciplinary team environment with several supervisors from different health care backgrounds (although you will still have a preceptor).

More importantly, your involvement in the APPE setting is likely to have a direct impact on patient care. No longer are you merely discussing theoretical patients with theoretical problems—this is the real thing. Although this may be intimidating, especially during your first few APPEs, you should consider your rotations an incredible opportunity to receive a form of hands-on training while under the guidance of more experienced health care professionals. Take advantage of this opportunity by being enthusiastic, motivated, hardworking, and prepared. Realize that the more effort you put into both your IPPE and APPE rotations, the greater your learning experiences.

## SELECTING AND SCHEDULING ROTATION EXPERIENCES

Experiential rotations provide a chance to develop your clinical skills in a relatively controlled environment before you become fully responsible for your own practice decisions. Therefore, carefully select your rotations. Talk with the OEE and your mentor early in your curriculum to get a good idea of which rotations can help provide exposure to different areas of pharmacy that will best fit you. In fact, you should be planning for your experiential training before the actual selection or assignment occurs.

In general, schools and colleges of pharmacy have required IPPEs and APPEs intended to provide the basic clinical skills and a well-rounded background to compliment and expand your didactic learning. Because these experiences are required, you will at most gain input relative to the timing and geographic location of specific activities. Assuming you have some input, schedule these required IPPEs and APPEs so they are least likely to interfere with desired APPE elective rotations that are highly competitive or available only at selected periods throughout your clinical year.

Your choice of APPE electives should be congruent with your longer-term career goals, at least to the extent you have developed such goals at this point in your career. For example, assume you plan to complete a postgraduate year one (PGY1) pharmacy residency program in an acute care hospital setting after graduation and then continue your training by completing a postgraduate year two (PGY2) specialized residency in emergency or critical care medicine. By taking one or two elective experiences in critical care and emergency medicine, not only will you build a solid foundation for your postgraduate training, but you will also meet preceptors who can be approached to provide letters of recommendation (see section on Letters of Recommendation).

## PRE-ROTATION PREPARATION

One useful way to prepare for either an IPPE or an APPE is to talk to students who have had the same experience in the not-too-distant past. The information these students can give you about the site, preceptor, and other health care personnel is often unavailable in the general description of the practice experience.

For example, ask the students what happens in a typical day, what responsibilities the preceptor assigns to students at the site, how and when evaluations are performed, and what they liked and did not like about the experience. You should be wary of extremely negative comments, particularly when they come from one student—as in statistics, sample size is important in proper data interpretation.

Another way to prepare for the experience is to contact the site preceptor a couple of weeks ahead of time using the contact method given to you by the OEE at your school or college. In addition to basic questions such as the time and place of your first meeting, you should ask whether you can do something to prepare for the experience such as reading key articles or guidelines pertinent to the area of practice. In addition, ask your preceptor if the site requires any special type of training or releases such as signed confidentiality statements and information system training for accessing patient health care information (e.g., EHR [electronic health record]). If several students are assigned to a particular site, preceptors may be able to perform this training as a group. Finally, let your preceptor know about any issues unique to you (e.g., medical conditions) that might require special consideration or accommodation in an experiential setting.

As you progress from your IPPEs to APPEs, your level of pre-rotation preparation should become more efficient and applicable to each specialized rotation.

## INTRODUCTION TO THE SITE

The first day at the site sets the stage for the remainder of the experience, so hopefully, you can contact your preceptor shortly before the rotation to schedule or coordinate a block of time on day 1 for an adequate orientation, which typically includes a tour of the facility and introductions to key personnel.

In general, your preceptor will realize that a few hours of dedicated time up front can prevent many potential problems and the need for an even larger time commitment in the future, particularly with IPPEs, and will be happy to set aside the few hours you request for day 1. If your preceptor is unavailable, perhaps another preceptor will be on-site who can assist in your orientation.

Personal characteristics of effective preceptors have been promulgated that can serve as model characteristics for students as well (Box 1) (Reference 11). Similarly, tips for effective precepting have been published (Box 2 and Box 3), many of which can be used by students to ensure that essential information is covered during the experience (Reference 12).

As a new student at the site, you should inform your preceptor of your past training and experiences, your personal goals and objectives for the rotation—which, of course, need to be reconciled with the rotation goals and objectives—and your future career goals. Also, ask the preceptor about any additional written or verbal information likely to be useful or needed for the experience (Box 3). By the time you begin your APPE rotations, the introductory period will likely be more succinct and more specific to the advanced experience.

### It's All About the Patient

The benefits that result from your provision of direct patient care are extended to the underserved areas of the experiential site and institution, the reputation of academic pharmacy programs (i.e., residency programs), and the efficiency of your preceptor (Reference 13). Providing direct patient care allows you to become more accountable and take a more active role in your own learning (Reference 13). Your involvement and pharmacy skill will help complete the site's tasks of providing a patient-centered medical home model, improving the quality of patient care, and reducing cost (Reference 14). By counseling your patients and engaging them in the decision-making care process, you, together with a team of health care providers, can improve clinical outcomes (Reference 14). Therefore, the patient should be the focus of your efforts in the experiential setting.

You achieve this patient-focused perspective by communicating with the patient. Because of the wide array of experiential settings and patient types, you should look to your preceptor for guidance during your first few patient encounters. He or she will be able to assist you with the logistics of the patient interaction such as the best time of day, the appropriate and relevant information, and, most importantly, how and where to document the interaction. Very few situations exist

**Box 1.** Characteristics of successful students (in no particular order).

- Passion for teaching and learning
- Ability to prioritize, integrate, and adapt
- Caring, respectful, and positive attitude
- Self-motivator (not procrastinator) with appropriate desire/ambition
- Team player with a win-win (not a win-lose) perspective
- Innovator with a desire to propose solutions, not just raise problems
- Skeptical, but not cynical, view when evaluating information
- Ongoing introspection with desire for self-improvement
- Desire to resolve minor problems before they become major problems
- Welcomes constructive criticism and makes improvements rather than dwelling on the negative aspects of the feedback

Adapted and reprinted with permission from the American College of Clinical Pharmacy. Originally published in Erstad BL. Surviving and thriving in the academic setting. In: Zlatic TD, ed. Clinical Faculty Survival Guide. Lenexa, KS: American College of Clinical Pharmacy, 2010:21-36 (Reference 11).

**Box 2.** Tips for effective preceptor-student interactions.

- Discuss and understand preceptor and student roles in experiential rotation.
- Maintain a friendly but respectful and professional relationship with your preceptor.
- Treat preceptor in the respectful manner you want to be treated.
- Model your preceptor's positive characteristics and behaviors.
- Define and personalize (to the extent possible) rotational goals/objectives.
- Understand your preceptor's expectations for your behavior and learning at the site.
- Assess and be assessed formally (midpoint, end) and informally (throughout) rotation.
- Use constructive feedback in your evaluations.
- Reinforce positive behaviors (e.g., professionalism).
- Help identify and resolve preceptor-student or team-student interaction problems.

Adapted and reprinted with permission from the American College of Clinical Pharmacy. Originally published in Erstad BL, Patanwala AE. Teaching and precepting: assuming the role of an educator. In: Murphy JE, ed. Resident Survival Guide. Lenexa, KS: American College of Clinical Pharmacy, 2011:53-68 (Reference 12).

**Box 3.** Examples of information discussed and/or provided to student.[a]

- Work Hours: Expected hours at site, restrictions on outside work responsibilities relative to those hours (if there is a potential interference), Board of Pharmacy restrictions (if applicable for your state)
- Contact Information: Routine and emergency contact information
- Orientation: General orientation information relative to specific site (ideally on day 1)
- Questions: How to answer the questions of other health professionals, particularly in the absence of preceptor (e.g., need to run all answers by the preceptor before making recommendations), handling potential problems that might arise (e.g., inability to reach preceptor in a timely manner)
- Health Care Team: Team composition (i.e., attending, resident, intern) and hierarchy (i.e., who you should approach with patient care issues), interactions with other trainees, pharmacists, and allied health professionals
- Daily Activities/Assignments: Integration and prioritization of activities, description of daily activities with handouts of information useful to patient care activities, expectations for patient case presentations (e.g., knowledge of medication uses, trade/generic names, dosing, route of elimination, adverse drug effects and interactions) including presentation format
- Patient Care: Responsibilities for care of patients and continuity of care when you are absent, patient confidentiality
- Administrative Activities: Expectations for meetings, rounds, conferences
- Medication Errors: Reporting potential or actual medication errors and adverse drug events
- Absences: Sick days, holidays, professional leave, and other days off
- Professionalism: Interactions and communications with other health care providers and patients, handling unprofessional behavior
- Assessment: Formal and informal evaluation process (set time aside with deadlines to complete each evaluation), inquire about formative (in progress) evaluations as well as summative (assessment at the end of experience) evaluations. Formative evaluations do not have to be formal written assessments, but rather, they more typically involve informal verbal feedback (see further discussion under Assessment).

[a]This list of items was originally published as a guide for preceptors, but it can be used to ensure that this type of information is conveyed to you during your experiential training.

Adapted and reprinted with permission from the American College of Clinical Pharmacy. Originally published in Erstad BL, Patanwala AE. Teaching and precepting: assuming the role of an educator. In: Murphy JE, ed. Resident Survival Guide. Lenexa, KS: American College of Clinical Pharmacy, 2011:53-68 (Reference 12).

in which some form of communication is not possible. Even patients on mechanical ventilators have an established mode of communication, like responding to questions by eye blinks (e.g., 1 blink for yes, 2 blinks for no) or finger or hand gestures. Particularly important times for medication-related patient discussions include: during patient hospital admission/discharge; during hospitalization when changes in medication regimens occur; and during any appointment in an ambulatory care setting. However, any opportunity to interact with patients should be viewed as a potential source of useful clinical information, a time to improve your patient communication skills, and a chance to serve as an ambassador for the pharmacy profession.

Try not to lose track of your patient-centered focus as you determine the optimal treatment regimens for your patients in an interdisciplinary care environment. Furthermore, do what you can to ensure continuity of care, regardless of whether this seems to be a priority for other members of your health care team. One final point: the more interactions with your patients, the better; however, in an interdisciplinary care setting, be careful not to give information to patients that might conflict with information given by your other health care provider colleagues. When in doubt, it is better to defer giving information to the patient until you have discussed it with other members of the health care team.

> *What we most wish we knew before starting rotations was how often we wouldn't know answers to questions and that we weren't expected to know the answers to all of them. However, we were still held responsible to look information up and be accountable for our own education.*
>
> —Joel Nielsen and Connie Chau, 2012 Pharm.D. graduates at University of Arizona, Tucson, Ariz.

## INTERDISCIPLINARY PATIENT CARE

Although the amount and mode of interaction between you and other health care professionals will vary somewhat from one experience to another, interdisciplinary practice with a patient focus is paramount in all practice settings. The need for interdisciplinary education and practice has been recognized by august groups like the Institute of Medicine (IOM) in their publication titled *Crossing the Quality Chasm: A New Healthcare System for the 21st Century* (Reference 15). Here, you will read the IOM recommendations for improving a patient's health care by focusing on safety and efficacy, as well as providing timely, efficient, and equitable patient-centered care (Reference 15). The IOM also suggests focusing on evidence-based practice when students are teaching and on providing students more opportunity for interdisciplinary training (Reference 15).

This IOM publication will assist in comprehending the complexity of the health care system and the many changes that would need to occur to change its direction (Reference 15). Nevertheless, the manner and extent to which interdisciplinary care is adopted and cultivated will likely vary from site to site during your experiential rotations. At one extreme, you may be immediately welcomed as an important member of the health care team, whereas at the other extreme, you may be asked why you are there and what you are supposed to do. With either extreme or something in the middle, you need to nurture your relationship with other team members, just as you do with your patients. You need to build rapport if it is not present, and maintain rapport if it is.

There are many ways to develop and sustain these interdisciplinary relationships, but one of the most important is face time. The more you interact with other team members to develop a trusting relationship, the more likely they are to encourage and implement your recommendations. Other ways to nurture this team relationship (beyond the previous discussions related to personal characteristics such as professionalism) include the following:

- Enthusiastically go beyond minimal expectations.
- Be a problem solver—Ask questions and help your team assess difficult cases; do not wait until you are asked a specific question before you begin researching a potential drug-related problem.
- Learn when to speak up—You may be the only person with certain information; however, you do not want to unnecessarily interrupt your team members.
- Remember that it is all about the patient, not about your getting credit for a recommendation or plan.
- Be proactive—Let team members know you are willing and able to help research and answer patient care questions.
- Anticipate problems or questions that might arise and have a well-researched response prepared ahead of time.

- When you are caught off guard by a difficult question from another team member, admit you do not know the answer and volunteer to find it.
- Try to foster team building, even if it means periodically helping with non-drug-related issues.

Research has shown that pharmacy students are potential contributors to both the clinical and economic benefits associated with patient care activities in the experiential setting (Reference 16). As a student in the experiential setting, you should realize that, in addition to your direct patient care responsibilities, you are an ambassador for pharmacy. When you perform admirably for your team and patients, the positive consequences of your efforts directly or indirectly reflect positively on the profession as a whole. Similarly, when you perform in a less-than-admirable manner, the negative consequences may be beyond your own reputation.

## Interdisciplinary Activities

Not all experiential rotations provide an opportunity for interdisciplinary rounds, but almost all rotations involve interactions with other health professionals in some manner, such as telephone conversations related to prescriptions. Your school or college of pharmacy will almost certainly include mock scenarios involving health care providers from various specialties. However, such interdisciplinary activities in various patient care settings have no true equivalent in the classroom, so you should do what you can to maximize the benefits from this experience, which will involve oversight from more experienced clinicians.

One of the first things you will learn in the experiential setting, if you have not learned it already, is that you will not know the answers for many of the questions raised by other health professionals. To make matters worse, as a relatively new practitioner, you will likely be surprised by the amount of knowledge your physician colleagues possess about medications, particularly medications commonly used in their area of practice. Therefore, when you are asked a question, it will often be a difficult one, for which you will not have a ready answer. Even when you think you have the correct answer to a clinical problem, you should realize that this is only the first step in a process that involves convincing and persuading other health professionals to implement your proposed solution.

It is important to keep in mind that proper, open communication between all members of the health care team results in better patient outcomes (Reference 17). Various methods of communication, both right and wrong, exist within the medical field. Methods to be avoided include using a condescending tone, failing to mention others' efforts, and blaming others for bringing faults to your attention (i.e., shooting the messenger) (Reference 17).

In general, some clinicians prefer a more direct approach, whereas others prefer a more subtle approach (e.g., bringing up the subject in a manner that makes them think they came up with the idea). Another approach is to ask a suggestive question or even a seemingly naive question (i.e., dumb question approach). Your preceptor should serve as a resource to provide insight on certain providers and methods of communication he or she uses that have been successful in building individual relationships. He or she can also give you advice on how to approach members of the team according to their rank within the institution (e.g., surgeon, physician assistant, second-year resident, medical student, nurse).

For example, if you are involved in caring for a patient who has been on an extended course of antimicrobial therapy that you believe is excessively long given the current literature, you could ask the clinician if there is a reason the patient is receiving therapy beyond the recommended number of days you found in a particular article or guideline. In some cases, you may interact with a clinician reluctant to adopt your solutions. This situation does not always have an easy answer. If you are interacting with a team involving other clinicians with decision-making authority, you may be better off taking your suggestions to them, assuming you can do so without alienating the reluctant clinician or breaking the protocol regarding who should be approached first in your particular clinical setting.

Perhaps one of the most frustrating situations you may encounter is being put on the defensive and having to end up trying to prove a non-provable proposition. For example, assume a clinician prescribes a dose of a medication that is not in any published literature obtained through a thorough search; furthermore, assume that no good theoretical basis exists for the medication dose. Thus, you question the order.

To your surprise, the clinician defends the order as is and asks you to "prove" the prescribed dose will not work better than the usual dose. You will be unable to prove the dose is wrong because you cannot prove a negative. For this reason, the affirmative team in formal debates has the obligation of proof because the affirmative team is tasked with proposing a solution different from the usual approach.

Similarly, it should not be incumbent on you as a student defending the traditional dose to prove the inappropriateness of the alternative dose. Of course, saying this is one thing, but dealing with this situation in an actual clinical encounter is likely to be much more nuanced and difficult and may require getting your preceptor or other, more experienced clinicians involved in the discussion.

Another situation you will likely encounter in the clinical setting that might lead to frustration is a clinician who elects not to take your medication-related recommendation. Rarely are medication-related decisions a simple dichotomous choice of this medication or that one. Often, there is more than one possible and reasonable option. Assuming this, you (and your preceptor) must decide when your recommendation warrants expending more than the usual time and effort to get it implemented. This situation is again context-specific and not amenable to a single solution.

### Case Scenario

A patient is receiving a proton pump inhibitor for prophylaxis of stress-induced bleeding when the patient could be receiving a somewhat less expensive histamine-2 antagonist with similar efficacy. You had planned to recommend a change to the latter therapy, but you know the physician prefers the proton pump inhibitor for his patients. To make things more complicated, assume you intend to make several other recommendations to the physician the same day with important patient safety implications. This is not the time to force the cost issue and risk not having your more important recommendations questioned. It is probably better to save the cost issue for a later date when other, more important decisions are not at stake. Handling situations such as this one requires the type of experience you gain through several encounters and variations in the clinical setting.

In health care, these situations are often referred to as using or not using evidence-based medicine. Throughout your experiential education and thereafter in your career as a pharmacist, you will commonly use evidence-based medicine to formulate your clinical decisions. Always be sure to perform thorough literature searches, appropriately analyze the data you find, and include patient-specific considerations such as health care access, insurance, total cost of the medication, and patient adherence.

### Interdisciplinary Rounding

If you are on a rotation that provides interdisciplinary rounding, there are a few additional issues to consider. You need to be prepared for rounds and always adhere to basic team etiquette: be professional and respectful, introduce yourself to those you have not previously met, be on time, and avoid interrupting someone presenting a patient case.

Before rounding, you should have had a discussion with your preceptor regarding medication-related resources that might be useful during rounds. A tertiary drug information resource, whether electronic or on hard copy, is likely to be needed, regardless of practice setting (see section on Resources). This will enable you to quickly retrieve information that does not require higher-level learning skills for proper interpretation, such as trade/generic names, FDA (U.S. Food and Drug Administration)-approved indications for use, dosage forms, and strengths. In your efforts to provide such information in a timely fashion, be careful not to look up answers to questions when you should be interacting with other team members in patient care discussions. Take advantage of the lulls in patient care activity to perform more extensive information searches, especially for difficult questions having answers your preceptor should check.

Team perceptions of pharmacy students vary from institution to institution and from physician to physician, so do not assume you will automatically be an accepted and valued member of the rounding team. Likely, you will have to earn your team's respect and confidence through proactive involvement in patient care activities.

Of importance, realize that the purpose of patient care rounds is to serve the immediate needs of the patient and that rounds are not always the best time to bring up care issues. In some cases, you will foster more of a collegial approach to patient care by bringing up potential problems in one-on-one conversations, possibly before or after the team rounds. Examples include potential medication-related problems less likely to have serious patient efficacy or safety concerns that likely occur because of simple oversight by a very busy physician in training. More in-depth learning and discussion of certain care issues might be most appropriate to discuss with your preceptor (see section on Patient Care Discussion with Preceptor). Bringing up several non-urgent patient care issues during busy rounds may not be the best use of the rounding time and may generate a low level of rapport with the team. *You should never make recommendations during rounds unless you are sure your information is correct.*

Gaining your team's trust will take some time and effort, and this trust could be quickly torpedoed by presenting questionable or, worse yet, inaccurate information. This usually means presenting your suggestions before rounds to your preceptor or another clinician supervising your training. Not only could an inappropriate recommendation harm the patient, it could also generate mistrust between you and your team that could hinder you during the remainder of the experience.

Especially during your early experiential rotations, you may feel frustrated because so many medication-related issues come up during rounds for which you have no answer. The best thing to do is state that you will look into the issue and ask how quickly the other health professional needs the information. Then, follow up in a timely manner with well-researched, accurate information that has been vetted by your preceptor or another clinician supervising your training. With this approach, the goal is for the team to recognize that you provide thoughtful and accurate patient care recommendations and ultimately involve you more in the decision-making process.

## PATIENT CARE DISCUSSIONS WITH PRECEPTOR

During the orientation to the rotation, you should have received guidance on the timing and expectations (e.g., format of presentation, information to be presented) for patient care discussions with your preceptor. These discussions can be very important to your learning and for providing optimal patient care. More informal patient care discussions are likely to occur when you interact throughout the day with a resident pharmacist or staff pharmacist. When rotations allow you to have more independent patient care activities, consider holding meetings with your preceptor that are more formal. In either case, you should be prepared for the discussions according to your preceptor's expectations and instructions. Typically, at minimum, this will include knowing the following information about your patients' medications:

- Trade and generic names
- Common indications
- Common and/or important adverse effects and/or interactions
- Usual dosing regimens
- Adjustments needed for hepatic or renal dysfunction

In addition, you will want to be able to present on your patients' disease state(s):

- Common findings and/or clinical presentation
- Guideline-based treatment regimens

Providing this type of information requires a relatively low-level form of learning (i.e., knowledge), and it is readily retrievable for most medications and disease states. If you have this baseline knowledge coming into the discussion, the conversation with your preceptor can be focused on more nuanced and higher-level learning. The bottom line for discussions with your preceptor is to be prepared.

## ASSESSMENT

Formative evaluations are intended to provide in-progress assessments of your learning during the rotation. In addition, there are usually less formal verbal evaluations of your progress toward achieving the stated goals and objectives of the experience. You should encourage such feedback from both your preceptor and other health care professionals who have substantial interactions with you at the site. For example, if you provide recommendations quite often to a certain physician, you should ask whether the information has been timely and useful; furthermore, you can ask what more you might do to improve the care of your patients. Although assessments in the experiential setting are often of this more formative nature and occur at episodic points throughout rotations, the need still exists for some type of summative evaluations, although different from the typical written testing used to assess learning in the classroom setting. You should view your experiential evaluations as another opportunity for learning. Therefore, you should request such feedback at the start of the rotation if there is any question whether it is routinely provided.

Hopefully, your preceptor will realize that assessments should be bidirectional and encourage you to provide similar formative and summative evaluations of his or her preceptorship. Usually, the summative evaluations of the preceptor by the student are mandated by the college through its experiential coordinator. Assuming this is the case, you should complete these evaluations in a constructive manner (i.e., evaluate your preceptor in the same professional way you expect the preceptor's evaluation of you to be performed).

## RESOURCES

As previously alluded to, many of the resources applicable for resident or preceptor development also provide important information for students during their experiential training. Furthermore, the student is encouraged to view the Web sites of national professional pharmacy organizations such the American Association of Colleges of Pharmacy and its companion journal, the *American Journal of Pharmaceutical Education*, both of which can be found at www.aacp.org. Along these lines, take advantage of opportunities at the local or state level (e.g., committees, task forces) pertaining to your development as a lifelong learner in pharmacy practice. For more information on integrating yourself into the pharmacy profession, see the chapter in this publication titled Step III: Get Involved.

It is difficult to give recommendations for more specific medication-related resources that apply to all experiential sites, other than a general drug information reference. If you have access to an electronic device that allows you to use various applications, you can ask your preceptor for recommended resources. Your preceptor will also be able to inform you of access to site-specific resources such as e-books or e-journals. As the number of clinical practice guidelines increases, one particularly useful Web site is www.guidelines.gov.

## LETTERS OF RECOMMENDATION

Displaying integrity in your work and committing to improve your patients' care will not only instill more self-confidence but will also offer greater preceptor satisfaction. This can lend you the ability to obtain a letter of recommendation from each preceptor you work with. If you are applying for postgraduate training or a clinical position, it is usually best to have at least two of your support letters from past or current (if sufficient time has passed) experiential preceptors. It can be beneficial to ask for letters from preceptors in your area(s) of interest. This way, the preceptor can comment not only on your work ethic and knowledge base, but also on your interest and passion for a certain area within pharmacy practice. It is important to ask your potential recommenders for permission to use them as references before listing them on your CV (curriculum vitae) or resume or before giving out their names to employers. Assuming they agree to write such letters, remember to follow up with a thank you.

## CONCLUSION

The experiential component of the curriculum can be one of the most challenging and rewarding aspects of your professional education. Adequate preparation for IPPE and APPE rotations will help ensure positive and productive experiences. Your attitude and behavior will play a critical role in your learning and effectiveness as a practitioner during each rotation. Constructive formative and summative evaluations during rotations should be used to enhance your pharmacy practice skills in a timely and effective manner. By maximizing every opportunity at each of your experiential practice sites, you will ultimately make a lasting impression on the pharmacy community and provide several stepping-stones for excelling in your future role as a pharmacy practice resident.

Box 4 summarizes many of the important points in this chapter for optimizing the chances of successful IPPE and APPE rotations.

**Box 4.** Important points for the experiential portion of the curriculum (Reference 1).

## Introductory Pharmacy Practice Experiences (IPPEs)
- Demonstrate an understanding of the basic concepts of ethical, professional, and legal behavior at all times.
- Develop the basic critical thinking and related clinical skills for general practice.
- Exhibit adequate and appropriate pre-rotation preparation.
- Ask basic rotation-related questions during your introduction to the site.
- Apply the basic concepts of interdisciplinary care to optimize the benefits and reduce the risks to the patients under your care.
- Provide a basic patient assessment with adequate knowledge of medications and disease states.
- Be able to appropriately analyze drug information and collect primary literature.
- Perform basic calculations for all medication doses, compounds, and pharmacokinetic evaluations.
- When team rounding is used at a site, demonstrate the appropriate way to raise important drug-related problems and respond to queries from other team members.
- Provide effective patient counseling at appropriate literacy levels by verbal, visual, and written communication methods.
- Be well prepared for discussions with your preceptor to ensure the optimal use of meeting times.
- Explain the differences between formative and summative evaluations, and tell how each should be used in a constructive manner to facilitate your learning during experiential rotations.

## Advanced Pharmacy Practice Experiences (APPEs)
- Demonstrate an understanding of more advanced context-specific concepts of professional, ethical, and legal behavior.
- Develop more advanced critical thinking and related clinical skills in more specialized areas of practice.
- Exhibit an advanced level of pre-rotation preparation.
- Be prepared to ask the focused questions needed to practice at the site during your introduction to the site.
- Demonstrate more advanced skills; for example, have your recommendations adopted in your role as an interdisciplinary team member.
- Provide a thorough patient assessment with a more complete knowledge of medications and disease states.

- Analyze literature and apply drug information to each specific patient case.
- Provide recommendations based on calculations of medication doses and pharmacokinetic profiles.
- When team rounding is used at a site, demonstrate a more nuanced and advanced level of interaction with other team members.
- Incorporate patients into their care with effective counseling and education techniques.
- Demonstrate a high level of preparation for discussions with your preceptor that optimizes your learning about the more nuanced aspects of more specialized rotations.
- Demonstrate how evaluations by your preceptor and other health care professionals can be implemented in a timely and efficient manner to improve your practice skills.

## ACKNOWLEDGMENT

*The authors would like to thank Pharm.D. graduates Joel Nielsen and Connie Chau for their thoughtful and constructive comments on this chapter.*

# REFERENCES

1. Accreditation Standards and Guidelines for the Professional Program in Pharmacy Leading to the Doctor of Pharmacy Degree. Tampa, FL: ACPE, February 2011.
2. American Pharmacists Association-Academy of Students of Pharmacy and the American Association of Colleges of Pharmacy Council of Deans. White paper on pharmacy student professionalism. J Am Pharm Assoc 2000;40:96-102.
3. Duke LJ, Kennedy K, McDuffie CH, Miller MS, Sheffield MC, Chisholm MA. Student attitudes, values, and beliefs regarding professionalism. Am J Pharm Educ 2005;69:Article 104.
4. Cain J, Scott DR, Akers P. Pharmacy students' Facebook activity and opinions regarding accountability and e-professionalism. Am J Pharm Educ 2009;73:Article 104.
5. Brown D, Ferrill MJ. The taxonomy of professionalism: reframing the academic pursuit of professional development. Am J Pharm Educ 2009;73:Article 68.
6. Brehn B, Breen P, Brown B, et al. An interdisciplinary approach to introducing professionalism. Am J Pharm Educ 2006;70:Article 81.
7. Poirier I, Gupchup GV. Assessment of pharmacy student professionalism across a curriculum. Am J Pharm Educ 2010;74:Article 62.
8. Hammer D. Improving student professionalism during experiential learning. Am J Pharm Educ 2006;70:Article 59.
9. Blouin RA, Riffee WH, Robinson ET, et al. AACP Curricular Change Summit Supplement: role of innovation in education delivery. Am J Pharm Educ 2009;73:Article 154.
10. Rathbun RC, Hester EK, Arnold AM, et al. Importance of direct patient care in advanced pharmacy practice experiences. Pharmacotherapy 2012;32:398.
11. Erstad BL. Surviving and thriving in the academic setting. In: Zlatic TD, ed. Clinical Faculty Survival Guide. Lenexa, KS: American College of Clinical Pharmacy, 2010:21-36.
12. Erstad BL, Patanwala AE. Teaching and precepting: assuming the role of an educator. In: Murphy JE, ed. Resident Survival Guide. Lenexa, KS: American College of Clinical Pharmacy, 2011:53-68.
13. Rathbun RC, Hester EK, Arnold AM, et al. ACCP Commentary: Importance of direct patient care in advanced pharmacy practice experiences. Pharmacotherapy 2012;32:e88-e97.
14. Larkin H. The patient-centered medical home. Trustee 2012;65:17-20.
15. Institute of Medicine. Crossing the Quality Chasm: A New Health System for the 21st Century. Washington, DC: National Academy Press, 2001.
16. Mersfelder TL, Bouthillier MJ. Value of the student pharmacist to experiential practice sites: a review of the literature. Ann Pharmacother 2012;46:541-8.
17. Ellison D. Build open communication for better patient care. Minn Med 2012;95:38-9.

# STEP VII
# EXPAND YOUR NETWORK

Keri A. Sims, Pharm.D., BCPS

## ABBREVIATIONS IN THIS CHAPTER

| | |
|---|---|
| APPE | Advanced Pharmacy Practice Experience |
| IPPE | Introductory Pharmacy Practice Experience |
| PGY1 | Postgraduate year one |
| PGY2 | Postgraduate year two |
| RPD | Residency program director |

You have heard the proverb, "it's not what you know, it's who you know." However, when it comes to obtaining the residency position of your choice, it is actually a combination of both. "What you know" can be defined as the knowledge and skills you learned throughout your pharmacy courses that essentially shaped you into a competent pharmaceutical care provider. "Who you know" is the network of professional contacts that can guide your residency search and write convincing letters of recommendation to help your application rise to the top.

## THE VALUE OF DEVELOPING A PROFESSIONAL NETWORK

The benefits of developing an extensive professional network are many. The most obvious benefit is the acquisition of persuasive letters of recommendation required for your residency applications. As you progress through pharmacy school, networking can also help you define your ideal career path, make educated choices regarding internships and externships, and identify mentors who will foster your professional development.

Pharmacy professionals or employers with whom you have had substantial, positive interactions (a.k.a. collaborators) or mentors are the prime candidates to write the letters of recommendation for your internship or residency applications. Early in your academic career, it may

**Table 1.** Timeline for Developing a Professional Network

| Professional Year | Recommended Networking Activities |
|---|---|
| P1 | - Take time to get to know your professors, employers, preceptors, and peers in the classroom, workplace, or within professional organizations.<br>- Use what you learn about different areas of pharmacy practice to set some potential short- and long-term career goals.<br>- Research summer internship opportunities.<br>- Seek out local pharmacy continuing education programs and/or a state pharmacy association meeting to attend. |
| P2 | - Continue to build and nurture professional relationships with professors, employers, preceptors, and peers.<br>- Continue your involvement in professional organizations and seek out leadership opportunities.<br>- Continue to define your career goals.<br>- Seek out summer internship opportunities.<br>- Attend a local or regional pharmacy meeting, if possible, and research whether you can attend a national meeting this year or next. Practice your networking skills at these meetings.<br>- Attempt to identify one or two individuals who could write a letter of recommendation for you if it were needed by the middle of the academic year. |
| P3 | - Continue to build and nurture professional relationships with professors, employers, preceptors, and peers.<br>- Actively pursue leadership opportunities within professional organizations.<br>- Continue to narrow and define your career goals.<br>- Identify shadowing opportunities, if needed, to help you determine your career goals or build your professional network.<br>- Attend a national meeting, if possible, and expand your network beyond your immediate geographic region.<br>- Identify whether any of your professional contacts have developed into a mentor for you. If so, continue to seek their guidance and assistance.<br>- By the end of the year, identify two or three individuals who will be able to write a letter of recommendation by December of your P4 year. |

| Professional Year | Recommended Networking Activities |
|---|---|
| P4 | • Continue to build and nurture your professional network.<br>• Make sure you are able to confidently express your career goals and display your abilities and past professional experiences.<br>• Make a strong effort to network at the national meeting(s) you attend.<br>• Contact the individuals you would like to have write letters of recommendation, and make sure they are comfortable writing a positive letter of recommendation for you. |

be difficult to identify several individuals who know you well enough to be able to serve as appropriate references; however, as you progress through pharmacy school, you will need to make a conscious effort to develop professional relationships in the classroom, on experiential rotations, at work, or through involvement in committees and extracurricular activities (see Table 1). If, by the end of your third professional year, you do not have at least two or three individuals who can write a convincing letter of recommendation, you should move professional networking up on your list of priorities.

You will likely need to interact with and learn from several pharmacists before you can define your ideal residency position or ultimate career path. Even the most casual conversation can open your eyes to additional ideas, details, and advice that will help you continue to establish your short- and long-term career goals. Don't be concerned if, early in your academic career, your definition of the ideal position changes frequently. It is perfectly normal to become enthusiastic about several different options. My personal career goal changed from association management to pharmaceutical industry to academia within just a couple of years of pharmacy school. One of the wonderful things about having a Pharm.D. degree is that you can take your career in several different directions.

In addition to helping you define your career goals, professional contacts can offer you advice specific to your institution. Perhaps there is a certain experiential rotation you should try to include in your schedule. Your interest in a field like critical care may be curtailed by not knowing the clinical pharmacist precepting the critical care rotation.

However, a faculty member with whom you have networked may be able to tell you that this particular pharmacist is a leader in the field and has been voted Preceptor of the Year. Likewise, your pharmacy school's faculty, administrators, upperclassmen, and classmates may provide you with information on available scholarships, internships, and research opportunities. Finally, is your institution unique in its approach to teaching pharmacy curricula? You can learn from your faculty and administrators how your institution's instructional methods differ from those in the rest of the country. You can also establish an ideal approach to explaining your institution's academic methods in an interview situation.

As you network and meet new people, you may be drawn to the advice of one person more than that of another. This attraction may be based on communication style, a shared common interest, or simply this person's ability to understand where you are and how to help you reach the next level professionally. It is important to recognize that as you continue to seek guidance from this individual, you are developing a mentoring relationship. A mentor is an experienced and trusted individual who invests in your professional development and is willing to offer you help and advice. A mentoring relationship may begin as a collaboration, in which an individual guides you through just one particular project like submitting and presenting your first poster presentation. If you continue to consult this individual throughout your career, he or she may become a mentor. It is common to have several different mentors according to your current location and particular needs. I have a mentor from whom I have sought advice for many years, yet the relationship began because of his strength—and my weakness—in statistics. I have another mentor whose strength is professional writing. Although I go to him first to edit anything I write, he has allowed me to call on him for guidance on both personal and professional issues that fall outside his expertise in professional writing but within his expertise of life experience and wisdom. Having mentors in your life will be critical to the success of your career.

## NETWORKING OPPORTUNITIES

Networking opportunities are all around you. You will find occasion to build professional relationships with peers, upperclassmen, faculty, and pharmacy practitioners on your school of pharmacy campus and

Colleagues - students

Professional contacts - faculty, employers, administrators, preceptors, other pharmacists

Collaborators - students, faculty, preceptors, employers

Mentors - faculty, preceptors, employers

Figure 1. Your professional network.

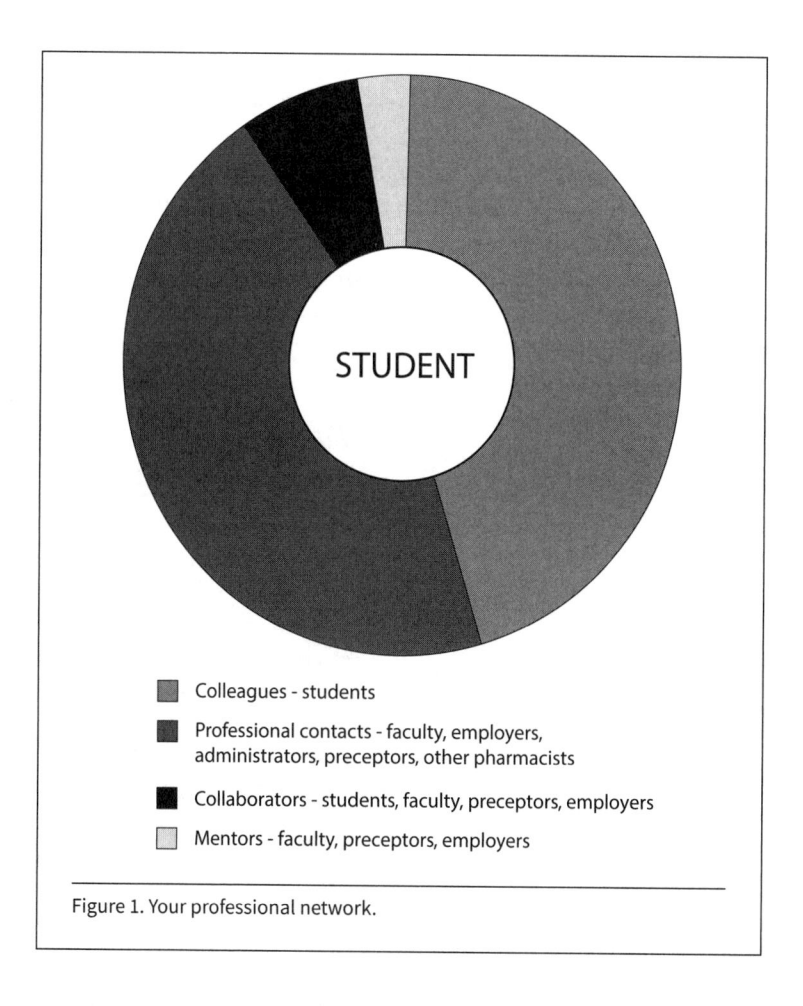

at your experiential sites. As you develop a professional network, pay close attention to its configuration. You will want to make sure you are developing a vast network of colleagues and contacts but are also taking the time to build more quality relationships with collaborators and a mentor or two (Figure 1).

## On Campus

You spend a lot of time on campus, so take advantage of the opportunity to expand your professional network by participating in classroom discussions and study groups and getting involved in extracurricular activities and professional organizations.

Your faculty can serve as important resources and contacts as you research residency programs. Therefore, it is important to intentionally interact with faculty both in and outside the classroom. Asking and responding to questions in the classroom can be excellent ways to make yourself known to your professor and peers. Asking well thought-out questions applicable to the lecture material can be beneficial to your classmates and may impress your professor. However, routinely asking silly questions or questions after the professor has lectured beyond the allotted time may prompt your classmates to let out a heavy sigh and roll their eyes when they see your hand go up. These questions can be taken up with the professor after class or during the professor's office hours. Whenever you communicate with faculty, you will want to make sure you do so in a professional manner. You can respectfully disagree with your professor, but you should avoid "burning bridges" by being disrespectful or unprofessional at any cost. This individual may have a practice site at which you desire to do one of your experiential rotations or perhaps he or she has completed 1 or 2 years of residency training at an institution to which you are considering applying. Your ability to maintain professionalism in all situations will allow faculty to speak highly of you and ease your progression to the next step on your career path. However, even one negative or unprofessional encounter can follow you and impede your ability to ultimately obtain a residency position.

> *Pharmacy is a very small world. If you're vocally negative about your program or a rotation, everyone will hear about it and everyone will talk about it. You don't want to be known as the negative pharmacy student. Expressing enthusiasm even over experiences you didn't enjoy as much gives a much better impression, and people are more willing to connect with and help students who are known to be engaged and enthusiastic. I tried to find at least one good thing about the rotations I didn't enjoy to use as talking points when I was asked instead of focusing on what I didn't like.*
>
> —Kirstin Kooda, 2012/13 PGY1 Pharmacy Practice Resident at Mayo School of Health Sciences, Rochester, Minn.

You also have the opportunity to develop relationships with your peers and upperclassmen as you spend time on campus studying, participating in extracurricular activities, or becoming involved in professional organizations. Do not underestimate the value of developing these relationships. Such relationships may benefit you in the very near future as an upperclassman secures a residency position at an institution you have your eye on. He or she will not only be able to offer you advice, but will also likely take part in interviewing the residency candidates the following year. His or her opinion, based on a multiyear relationship with you, may be considered by the residency program director (RPD).

Currently, your peers may appear to be competition for you, but be confident in your own skills and encourage your classmates. You may continue to cross paths with them throughout your career. Someday, you may find yourself looking to change geographic locations, and a classmate in the area could be a precious resource for job opportunities.

The benefits of getting involved with extracurricular activities and professional organizations are vast and are detailed in Step III: Get Involved. More importantly, this involvement will allow you to network outside your campus community and begin reaching out to more pharmacy practitioners and RPDs.

## Experiential Sites

Your Introductory and Advanced Pharmacy Practice Experience (IPPE, APPE) preceptors will not only provide you with hands-on training, but can also serve as valuable resources when it comes to expanding your professional network. Your IPPE preceptors will help you define your career goals and point you in the right direction to pursue them. Your ability to impress your preceptor early in your academic career will lead to additional opportunities, possibly in the form of professional advice, research projects, or employment openings.

However, APPE preceptors have an even greater impact on your pursuit of postgraduate training. During a 4- to 6-week rotation period, your APPE preceptor knows not only how prepared you are for your daily duties and larger projects, but also whether you come in early, leave early, and dress appropriately, as well as whether you get along well with others at your site. By the end of the rotation, your preceptor has a solid assessment of your current abilities and potential to excel. Your preceptor is able to evaluate your attitude toward being challenged and learning new information and skills. Therefore, it is of utmost importance to make the most of your experiential educational opportunities (see Step VI: Maximize Experiential Education). In addition to writing letters of recommendation, preceptors can help guide you through researching residency programs and applying for residency positions. However, be aware of the timeline in the residency application process (see Step X: Step Up to the Plate: Bringing It Home in Your Final Professional Year). You will complete the application process in January. Therefore, design your APPE rotation schedule to allow time to develop significant relationships with the preceptors you have in mind to write letters of recommendation.

In addition to your primary preceptor, you will have the opportunity to impress and learn from others at your APPE rotation site. There may be several preceptors and pharmacy residents at your site. Take advantage of opportunities to cross paths and interact with these individuals. If you are struggling with a project or question from a physician, you can approach these individuals for help. Likewise, you can volunteer to help simply by saving a seat for someone at a lecture or even help collect patient information for a research project. Every effort to be part of the team will be noticed and will help you build several professional relationships. As you build these collegial relationships, you will continue to learn new information that will be of help to you in defining your career goals and devising a strategy to achieve them. Perhaps you will hear about an incredible residency program that matches your career goals and geographic preference while having lunch with a new colleague in the hospital cafeteria.

### Professional Meetings

Professional meetings are networking havens. If you attend a professional meeting and do not meet someone new, pay close attention to the following section on the nuts and bolts of How to Network. As you have the opportunity to attend state and regional professional meetings, your networking opportunities will abound. Typically, these meetings, which are not overwhelming in size, provide many opportunities for interacting with students, faculty, and pharmacists outside your city and school of pharmacy. By contrast, although national pharmacy organization meetings provide networking opportunities with students and pharmacists from across the country, it is easy to become overwhelmed by the sheer number of individuals in attendance. Taking the time to plan your meeting agenda will help make national pharmacy meetings more manageable and beneficial. For example, a student interested in pursuing residency training and a future career as a cardiovascular pharmacy specialist in the state of Texas will design his or her meeting experience to include student-specific programming, educational sessions and poster/platform presentations on cardiovascular topics, and possibly a state of Texas networking reception. In doing so, the student will meet others with similar interests, including residency preceptors. In addition, as you attend programming and events that meet your needs year after year, you will begin to see the same individuals on a consistent basis and strengthen your professional relationship with them.

Networking opportunities at professional meetings will present themselves in the form of breakfasts, lunches, receptions, or meetings. Any time food or drink is served at a professional meeting, you will likely have the opportunity to meet new people. Be sure to review the meeting's schedule and include these types of networking events in your personal itinerary. Avoid opting out of a breakfast designed to put you in touch with other professionals in your quest to get more sleep. In addition, during meeting sessions, rather than sitting next to your classmate or faculty member, consider sitting next to someone you do not know. Take the initiative to introduce yourself and learn more about this individual. The advantage of being a student at these meetings is that you are very likely to meet someone with more pharmacy experience than you have. If you happen to meet a fellow student, consider how his or her network and knowledge base is different from yours and whether it is therefore beneficial to add him or her to your growing list of professional contacts.

Poster presentations are another important networking opportunity. If you are presenting a poster, you will have the chance not only to meet professionals interested in your topic, but also to impress them with your research and communication skills. If you are not presenting a poster, you can attend the poster session and seek out posters that are within your therapeutic areas of interest. You will then have the opportunity to display your critical thinking skills by asking well thought-out, intelligent questions of the poster presenter. If a poster presenter does not remember you the next time your paths cross, you can refer back to the research presented to develop a common ground for future conversation.

Similar to poster presentations, you will have the opportunity to attend educational programming specific to your interests. Not only will you gain pharmacy knowledge, but you will also learn who are considered thought leaders in a particular field of study. Place these names and faces into your memory bank or networking file. You will then know whom to approach at a reception, as well as have their presentation to reference during your conversation.

You may or may not be familiar with a curbside consult. This occurs when a physician informally asks a colleague in another specialty for the best method of managing a particular clinical problem (Reference 1). As a pharmacy student, you may encounter many formal networking opportunities at professional meetings, but some of the most valuable of these are curbside in nature. Do you know the person beside you in the convention center elevator or at the hotel fitness center? Did you meet the person next to you also waiting for a table at a nearby restaurant or for transportation to the airport? When attending a large meeting, your odds of striking up a conversation with another pharmacist are pretty good. It may produce nothing more than casual conversation, or your effort to be outgoing may introduce you to several contacts, together with opportunities to prove your communication skills and professional development. These curbside encounters may also occur at places other than the areas surrounding a national pharmacy meeting. I recently met a visitor at my church (in Wisconsin) who happened to be a postgraduate year one (PGY1) resident applying for postgraduate year two (PGY2) programs. She informed me of the PGY2 programs she was applying to. I was able to highly recommend one of the RPDs (in Georgia). This RPD once taught me in pharmacy school (in Iowa), and I have had more recent interactions with her through my work with the American College of Clinical Pharmacy (ACCP). I greatly doubt that the PGY1 resident thought she would have a networking opportunity at church that morning.

## Shadowing

If you feel you have not had adequate opportunities to build a professional network or learn about a particular career path, you can seek out shadowing opportunities. A professor or administrator (e.g., dean, associate/assistant dean, department chair) within your institution may be able to put you in touch with a clinical pharmacist practicing in a therapeutic area that interests you. You will need to take the initiative to contact the pharmacist and see if you can set up a day or half-day to shadow him or her. Shadowing experiences provide you the opportunity to observe clinical pharmacy practice and to be a "fly on the wall." However, use discernment regarding when the pharmacist and environment will allow you to ask questions. At that time, be prepared to display professional communication and critical thinking skills in the questions you ask. I had the opportunity to observe open heart surgery during one of my internships. It is not an appropriate time to ask questions when standing over an open chest next to a surgeon holding a heart in his hands. Rather, waiting for cardiology rounds to resume while shadowing a cardiac clinical pharmacist could be an ideal time to ask questions.

## HOW TO NETWORK

As networking opportunities present themselves, some people are more natural communicators and socializers than are others. You may have a natural curiosity about people and hardly be able to keep questions from jumping out of your mouth, whereas others' minds may go completely blank after an initial introduction. Therefore, the first step is to determine where you fall on this communication continuum. Once you have assessed your natural communication abilities, you can determine how much effort and preparation you will need to invest in before attending any planned or informal networking opportunity.

### Planned Networking Opportunities

Regardless of your natural communication skills, it is always wise to have a strategy when attending planned networking opportunities like professional meetings. First and foremost, always be prepared to state your short- and long-term professional goals. One method for doing so is to prepare a 60-second statement that fully encompasses your goals. Write this statement as a bullet point list, and rehearse it in front of the mirror. You will want to make sure it sounds as good "live" as it does in your head. Second, you want to think about who may be present at this networking event and if there is anyone you would like to meet. If you are at a regional conference, are you looking for representatives from a particular institution? At a national meeting, are you hoping to meet someone from a geographic location to which you hope to relocate or leaders in a specific therapeutic area? Finally, articulate a few thoughtful, yet general questions in advance that you can easily access as needed. If your career goals are still very general, your strategy can be general as well. A plan to meet and learn from at least five new individuals is a solid course of action.

Once you've developed your strategy to a planned networking event like a reception, prepare to be assertive and confident without being pushy or aggressive. Make sure that your firm handshake, ability to look people in the eye, business card, and appearance are ready to make a positive impression. Avoid interrupting conversations, but take advantage of a lull in the conversation to introduce yourself to someone new. Many times, someone you already know (a faculty member or mentor) will introduce you to someone new. Typically, this will occur naturally, but it is appropriate to ask them to introduce you. Then, you may benefit from the domino effect: that new contact will introduce you to an additional person and so on.

Once introduced, be prepared with a few general questions. If you don't already know, you can ask new contacts what type of pharmacy practice they are involved in, where they trained, or how much they are involved with students or residents. In asking these types of questions, you are searching for some common ground with these individuals. Once you discover that you share an acquaintance, interest in a particular study, or even a hobby, the conversation will flow more easily, and the individual is more likely to remember you.

On occasion, the search for common ground with new contacts may fail. At that point, you have two options. First, you can continue to ask questions and learn about the individual. This is a kind gesture; however, you risk leaving a bad impression if the conversation becomes strained. Second, you can politely excuse yourself from the conversation. It is best to avoid making up a reason like "If you'll excuse me, I need to meet my professor at 7 p.m." Rather, say "It was very nice meeting you; thank you for taking the time to talk with me." Although it may be difficult to exit a one-on-one conversation, it is best to avoid being caught in a lie.

In general, listen more than you speak, but take advantage of the chance to promote yourself. You want to continue to seek advice from your network, so ask a lot of questions. However, you can ask your questions in ways that display your experiences and skills. For example, "When I interned at Children's Hospital, I found that most clinical pharmacists were very active in research. Is that how it is at your institution?" This conversation will teach you about the role of research within clinical pharmacy positions at a different institution and allow you to highlight your main internship projects.

You may have moments when you feel that you missed an opportunity. For example, perhaps you didn't meet the person you wanted, forgot to ask a question, or failed to subtly promote yourself. All of those things are expected to happen, but it is good to start networking early to ensure you have many opportunities to build your network throughout your academic career.

Meeting and conversing with new professional contacts are the first two factors in expanding your network through planned networking events. However, the third factor is remembering whom you met and what you talked about. Make every effort to remember the names of your new contacts. Consider developing a file (paper or electronic) that includes the person's name, title, institution, and your common interests. When you have time, you can use the Internet to make sure you have the name spelled correctly and add other pieces of information to your file like photos and key publications. The concern is not that you would offend someone if you forgot the specifics of his or her presentation; rather, you want to use what you learned from that individual to impress him or her on your second meeting. The easiest and most crucial things to remember are the common ground you found, as this will be how the person remembers you. But don't be offended if they don't remember you. You can still say something like, "I met you last year at this meeting. I'll never forget that you advised me to shadow someone in pediatric oncology since my school doesn't offer a rotation in it. Thank you. That was very helpful advice." Most likely, the two of you will now have plenty in common to converse about, and hopefully, your new professional contact will continue to offer you valuable advice, such as which PGY1 programs also offer a particular PGY2 specialty program within the same institution. You can even send important new contacts a short note, stating that it was nice to meet him or her and that you look forward to your next meeting.

## Informal Networking Opportunities

Informal networks develop naturally as you pursue your studies and live in your community. Your informal network may be defined as your colleagues and collaborators who have had the opportunity to work with you. Your ability to communicate your professional goals and ask questions to find common ground is still very important to developing an informal network. However, the need to move gracefully through a formal reception is not nearly as critical as working hard and displaying integrity. Can people depend on you to arrive on time, be prepared, meet deadlines, strive for excellence, and work well with others? The reputation you build for yourself as you progress through your pharmacy curriculum is extremely important. If your reputation is good, opportunities to be involved and even lead will continue to present themselves, and you will have plenty of individuals willing to write glowing letters of recommendation. If you have done something to tarnish your reputation, like fail to show up for an exam or an event you were to play a significant role in, you don't have to completely give up all hope for acquiring a residency position. It is possible to repair a burnt bridge. You are human, and you will make mistakes. If you are guilty of such an incident, you cannot simply sweep it under the rug and hope it disappears. Rather, you should approach the person you failed or offended and apologize. You will need to convince the individual that you have matured and will not be guilty of such an offense again. Most likely, he or she will respect your sincere efforts to right a wrong and give you a second chance. However, your efforts will have to be sincere, as you will not likely get a third chance.

## E-PROFESSIONALISM

A chapter on networking would be amiss if it did not include online social networking. A study of health professional students' (including pharmacy students) use of social media found that of the 644 first-year students surveyed, 77% used Facebook (Reference 2). There are potential professional benefits to using social networking sites. They can help you maintain correspondence and share ideas with classmates, upperclassmen, and new professional contacts. However, the rules of professionalism that apply to the interview scenario apply to all professional correspondence, be it live, by e-mail, or posted to the Internet through Facebook, LinkedIn, Twitter, YouTube, or even a blog. Therefore, you must maintain an account of the highest standard of professionalism. This includes photos you are tagged in and what others contribute to your page, as well as your outgoing comments. You are creating a permanent record when you post to the Internet. Many employers and schools of pharmacy do Internet searches before hiring or interviewing candidates. Therefore, everything that is tied to you should be appropriate to share during an interview situation.

Your efforts to safeguard your name are a worthwhile step in building a competitive residency application. As a test, try to find out as much as you can about yourself using the Internet. What comes up when you Google your name? Is your Facebook profile picture appropriate to show to a professional audience? Ensure that your name is not connected to any unprofessional behavior.

In general, it is not recommended to "friend" faculty, preceptors, RPDs, residency preceptors, or patients (References 3, 4). Refraining from this will help maintain professional boundaries. If you receive a "friend" request from a faculty member or professional networking contact, it is preferred that you decline the invitation and maintain correspondence through other channels.

## CONCLUSION

A decision to pursue pharmacy residency training will take you down a career path in clinical pharmacy—a world that is even smaller than the world of pharmacy. You will continue to cross paths with classmates, faculty, colleagues, and preceptors as you progress through your career. The relationships you develop throughout your career will benefit you personally and professionally.

Taking the initiative to expand your professional network now, as a student, will not only provide you with extra guidance to define your career goals, but also put you in touch with the professionals who can help you achieve those goals. Your efforts to strive for excellence in your schoolwork, show integrity in extracurricular activities, display your abilities on experiential rotations, and take advantage of networking opportunities will allow faculty, mentors, and professional contacts to confidently recommend you as an outstanding residency candidate.

## REFERENCES

1. Diamond C. Access to specialty care. N Engl J Med 1995;332:474.
2. Giordano C, Giordano C. Health professions students' use of social media. J Allied Health 2011;40:78-81.
3. Chretien KC, Farnan JM, Greysen SR, Kind T. To friend or not to friend? Social networking and faculty perceptions of online professionalism. Acad Med 2011;86:1545-50.
4. Metzger AH, Finley KN, Ulbrich TR, McAuley JW. Pharmacy faculty members' perspectives on the student/faculty relationship in online social networks. Am J Pharm Educ 2010;74:Article 188.

# STEP VIII
# ENGAGE IN RESEARCH AND SCHOLARSHIP

Jerry L. Bauman, Pharm.D., FCCP, FACC

## INTRODUCTION

After my consistently disastrous performances in organic chemistry lab during pre-pharmacy, I entered pharmacy school with the intent of *not* pursuing any form of what I considered research during my upcoming pharmacy education or career. Rather, I wanted to be a practicing pharmacist. It was not until my senior year in pharmacy school that I realized that I could actually do both and that perhaps research and scholarly activities were not as repugnant as I had once thought.

During my senior year in pharmacy school, I met several of the new clinical faculty at the University of Illinois and was fortunate enough to be subsequently accepted into the residency after graduation. Early in my residency, there was a back-and-forth controversy in the *New England Journal of Medicine* (a journal I had begun reading) regarding whether phenytoin solution could safely be added to intravenous fluids for administering to patients. So, after a discussion with my preceptor, we added some Dilantin to a single bag of 5% dextrose, and voila—an explosion of crystals, plain to see. But were they phenytoin? We filtered the bag and collected the crystals; then, with the help of my medicinal chemistry professor, we did a simple melting point determination: they were indeed phenytoin. With this very simple experiment and n=1, I wrote a letter to the editor of the *New England Journal of Medicine* (Reference 1). Several weeks later, I received a letter accepting my small contribution. I was instantly hooked! What fun, how exciting—but also rather scary. My residency project that year was built on this initial simple experiment. We designed a study to examine the stability of phenytoin solution in a variety of intravenous fluids and discovered it to be relatively stable in saline (but not dextrose), and using the dreaded Henderson-Hasselbalch equation (which I was made to memorize at least 35 separate times during pharmacy school but never actually used), we also discovered why this is so. The subsequent publication (Reference 2) was verified by other papers, and clinicians began routinely administering phenytoin as an admixture to saline piggybacks rather than using the troublesome intravenous push or intramuscular routes. My work solved a nuisance clinical problem and changed clinical practice in a small way. I certainly did not find the cure for cancer with this research, but it was so very personally rewarding. Because of these initial experiences during my student and residency years, I knew right then that I wanted to pursue clinical research and publish my ideas and results, in addition to practicing clinical pharmacy.

As I just illustrated, scholarship and research can be personally rewarding and fun, and it can actually help patients—so why else would you choose to pursue this during your Pharm.D. program? First, several pragmatic reasons exist for doing so. As everyone knows, matching into a PGY1 pharmacy residency is highly competitive these days. In addition to a strong academic record, you need impressive letters of support and recommendations from clinical faculty. Developing a strong professional relationship with one of these individuals surrounding a research or scholarly project will obviously facilitate this type of support and could provide a lasting mentor for your career. Many exceptional pharmacy students are competing for residency slots, and program directors look for distinguishing features in an applicant. Adding research experience, presentations, abstracts, and papers to your resume will certainly be noticed and valued. These activities help set you apart from the masses: initiating and completing a research project shows residency directors that you have the diligence and perseverance to start a project and see it through to completion. All of these are highly desirable traits in residents, and this is an excellent way for students to directly show they have these qualities. According to the accreditation standards, completion of a "practice-related project" is a required component of a postgraduate year one (PGY1) residency. Completion of "pharmacy practice research" can be used as an elective in a PGY1 residency. Thus, experience in this regard during your pharmacy school years will clearly aid your performance during the residency. This will be appreciated by those making decisions for the match. Second, there are many altruistic reasons to pursue research during your Pharm.D. education. Simply put, the skills you acquire in the conductance of the project will help you in your future career growth. I always recommend that our students develop a habit of contributing in a scholarly way throughout their career. Lecturing at local or national professional meetings, presenting posters of practice projects, publishing papers in journals, and pursuing other scholarly endeavors will increase your visibility and, frankly, your marketability. The skills you acquire during the Pharm.D. program will aid in your success as you progress through your career. Finally, publishing scholarly works actually helps your clinical practice. You personally reap the recognition that accompanies the scholarly contribution, and (sometimes all of a sudden and rather surprisingly) you are viewed as an "expert" in the field. Other pharmacists and health care practitioners seek your counsel in that area. In addition, if the paper was done in collaboration with others such as physicians, extremely helpful professional relationships are sometimes created. All of these outcomes—the results of completed and impactful scholarship—will aid in your effectiveness as a clinical pharmacist. In a recent study, almost 90% of students who were required to complete a P4 research project believed it provided a competitive advantage for postgraduate job opportunities (Reference 3). Furthermore, students who were specifically seeking a residency or fellowship were even more likely to see the value in this activity.

What do I mean by scholarship and research? Officially, most follow the definitions of Boyer (Reference 4), who broadly categorized scholarship in a variety of forms. Examples are the scholarship of application (i.e., clinical practice) and the scholarship of engagement (i.e., public service). Research is the *scholarship of discovery*. A few Pharm.D. programs require a research or scholarly project for graduation, but most do not. So, unless you are currently at one of those colleges, you will likely have to pursue this on your own. I recommend that you engage in a project that may be broadly shared with others and that the information therein be disseminated in some format. In other words, the fruits of your labor should have a result such as a presentation to a national or regional meeting or publication in a professional journal. This method will help you pursue projects that others want to learn about, and it will look better on your curriculum vitae (CV). So how would you go about this?

## STEPS OF A RESEARCH PROJECT
### Identify an Issue/Question to Study/Answer
I'm certain that, every day during your clerkship experiences (it could be during IPPE [Introductory Pharmacy Practice Experience] or, more likely, APPE (Advanced Pharmacy Practice Experience), when you are completely immersed in patient care activities), you and your preceptor

are confronted with drug therapy problems in which the solutions are unknown. In my career, almost every research idea I ever had resulted from observations (and frustrations) made in my clinical practice. Therefore, be observant during your rotations (Figure 1 and Figure 2). Some are big problems and big unknowns, and some are small problems. A big question may be whether to recommend aspirin to a patient with hypertension and high cholesterol but without end-organ damage from those disorders. Of course, solving this question would require thousands of patients with many centers and investigators, which is not feasible for you. Moreover, solving big problems requires big budgets, and you are broke; Pharm.D. students should not be required to write grants to get their ideas funded or be solely responsible for obtaining funding for the project. Nonetheless, assisting your mentor in preparing a grant can be a great experience and helpful in years to come. Pharm.D. students have opportunities to compete for small awards (e.g., the American Foundation for Pharmaceutical Education [www.Afpenet.org], other professional societies). Because of these challenges you will encounter, my advice to you during your Pharm.D. years is to stick to a small problem (save the big ones for when you are a famous professor later on) with a modest cost. In fact, if you plan to begin and complete the project, any question that requires the prospective recruitment of patients to enter the study will frankly be difficult to complete. Some faculty mentors will recruit and use Pharm.D. students (or residents) sequentially; in other words, you may be asked to help with an ongoing study, and your predecessor and successor may work on other parts. Although this approach can indeed provide valuable experience, you will miss the complete experience of the study, from

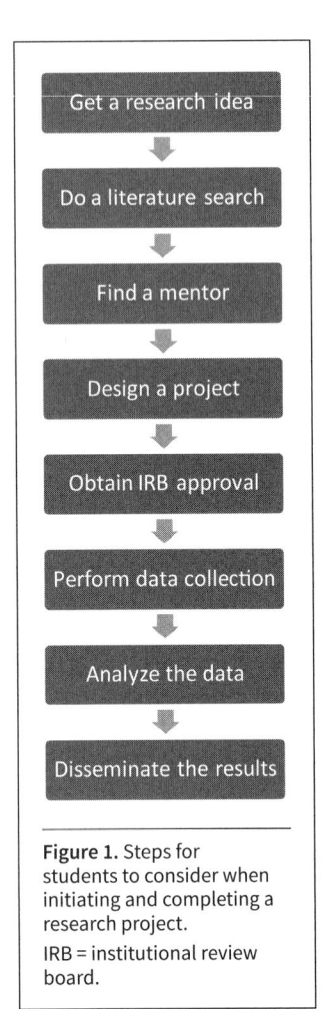

Get a research idea
↓
Do a literature search
↓
Find a mentor
↓
Design a project
↓
Obtain IRB approval
↓
Perform data collection
↓
Analyze the data
↓
Disseminate the results

**Figure 1.** Steps for students to consider when initiating and completing a research project.
IRB = institutional review board.

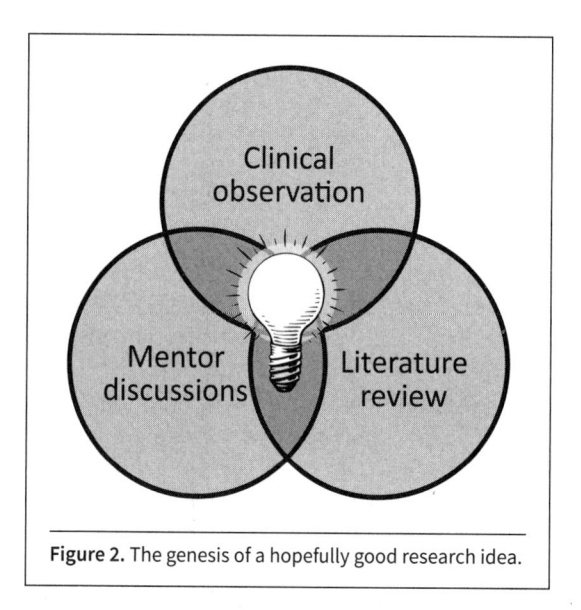

Figure 2. The genesis of a hopefully good research idea.

generating the hypothesis to presenting the results. Therefore, I usually recommend that students think small and doable in a relatively short period. Examples of these types of studies or contributions to consider (retrospective chart reviews, in vitro experiments, case reports) will be reviewed later in this chapter. One last piece of advice in choosing a topic of study: pick one that is interesting to you and that stimulates your curiosity. It's much more fun to discover something about which you are passionate or interested in.

## Do an Exhaustive Literature Search on the Topic and Read Everything You Can About It

If you plan to disseminate your results, you have to become an expert in the area. Therefore, you must become intimately familiar with all the published reports on the subject. Why haven't others considered attempting your planned study? More than once, I have had a potential research idea only to find that others had the same idea (there are many smart folks out there), and the original question had already been answered. You certainly don't want to be embarrassed to find out later (e.g., during manuscript submission or presentation at a meeting) that others have already published very similar findings or that you overlooked their studies. Look for areas in the topic that have not been fully explained or studied so that you can make a unique and valued contribution. Replicating someone else's work may provide valuable verification, but there is far greater impact in finding something new. However, just as often, you may be surprised by the small issues that have not been fully explored. It's in that niche that you want to design your experiment.

### Find a Faculty Mentor

Faculty members in colleges of pharmacy are extremely diverse, ranging from very basic scientists (medicinal chemists, pharmacologists, drug delivery, etc.) to applied pharmaceutical scientists (translational scientists, outcomes research, clinical trials, etc.). It is assumed that your intent is to acquire research skills in the more applied areas. Though having basic laboratory research experience (and publications or presentations) on your CV may help in other career options, I'm uncertain whether it will help you in your residency quest (although it will be helpful if you are considering laboratory research after completing the residency). Do your homework when approaching a faculty member to act as your mentor for a research or scholarly project. Clinical faculty members will have areas of specialty and expertise; obviously, you would like to match your area of interest with theirs. Furthermore, and particularly with the recent explosion of new schools of pharmacy, the research and scholarly abilities of the clinical faculty member may vary considerably. Someone with a record of scholarly contributions would be optimal; someone with no publications, not so. A quick literature search (e.g., PubMed) of your potential faculty mentor's publications will show both his/her area of interest and his/her publication record.

Clinical faculty members in colleges of pharmacy are generally on a "tenure track" or a nontenure track. Those on a tenure track have required scholarly responsibilities as a prerequisite to their continued employment, so these individuals tend to be more research-intensive. Nevertheless, many nontenure-track faculty have substantial scholarly responsibilities (required for academic promotion, though they may not be required for continued employment), and they tend to have more patient care duties (where the ideas come from!). More than likely, you will secure a mentor for your project simply by being assigned to that mentor's rotation during your Pharm.D. program. Moreover, the aforementioned project idea will have more than likely arisen during conversations surrounding patient care between you and your preceptor. Most clinical faculty (tenure track or nontenure track) eagerly pursue (or should) scholarly projects because they are academically rewarded for such contributions. In turn, they will (or should) be open to your invitation to assist you and willing to serve in this role. Developing the professional relationship between you and your mentor could prove to be a valuable and long-lasting one; this individual will more than likely serve as a reference for your application to residencies and perhaps job opportunities thereafter. In addition, they will hopefully have some discretionary funds at their disposal to help pay for the project.

## Design a Small Project and Write a Research Protocol

A written research protocol should always be prepared, even if the project does not need approval by the institutional review board (IRB). The protocol should include a hypothesis, background (literature review) on the issue, and clearly stated purpose of the study. It should also include specific and detailed methodology; anticipated methods for data analysis, including statistics; and anticipated findings and their potential significance or impact. Potential obstacles should be anticipated. This protocol serves not only as an important guide but also as an official record of your planned work. In addition, it forces you to carefully consider all the steps and issues surrounding the research in a written way. Because there are time constraints of performing a potentially publishable project during your Pharm.D. education, what types of projects might you consider? Allow me to provide some examples of the types of simple research projects appropriate for a Pharm.D. student, from my own experience.

### *Retrospective Case Series*

Perhaps you witnessed an unusual adverse effect of a specific drug during your experiential rotation or observed a peculiar method of administering a drug. On reviewing the literature, you found a paucity of published information on this subject. For example, we published a study about a series of patients with rapid supraventricular arrhythmias who had received continuous-infusion verapamil to slow their ventricular rate (Reference 5). This small study, completed with the assistance of a Pharm.D. student, showed proof of concept (i.e., that continuous infusion of intravenous calcium blockers could be easily titrated to control ventricular rate in arrhythmias such as atrial fibrillation), which eventually led to an accepted method of practice for other, similar drugs (diltiazem). We were doing this on a clinical basis to treat patients, and it was the Pharm.D. student's idea to share this experience (through publication) with others. As another example, we observed a torsades de pointes case caused by quinidine that occurred years after the patient was initially started on quinidine; the patient had tolerated it very well up until this life-threatening adverse effect. How unusual—why would this suddenly happen? We decided to collect and analyze all the cases of quinidine-induced torsades de pointes in our hospital database and those that we had collected through another study. What we found was that in almost all of these "late" instances of torsades de pointes caused by quinidine, there was another, more recent occurrence that could have further lengthened repolarization (QT interval) (Reference 6). It was as if these factors were additive (which we suggested in the published paper), and collectively, they caused torsades de pointes. These findings and those of others led to the concept of repolarization reserve in the occurrence of acquired torsades de pointes. In both examples, the ideas for the project were born of clinical observations during experiential rotations with trainees such as Pharm.D. students and residents, and both were published with some degree of impact on patient care. Moreover, both were doable in a reasonable timeframe. Both required approval by the IRB to review patient records, but they required "expedited review" as opposed to full review, which also saved time. This form of scholarship can be described as retrospective "observational" and is not highly hypothesis driven (i.e., you are just observing what has happened naturally, so to speak; there is no intervention). The scope of these projects can vary. The investigator might collect a small series of patients in a single database, as in the examples shown, or if access is possible, the investigator might collect many cases from large multicenter data sets. Pharmacoepidemiologic studies can be entirely observational, in which the investigators passively and retrospectively observe the effects of a treatment on a disease (for example) in large data sets.

*Analysis of Already Existing Data*
Some forms of research studies rely solely on existing data, obviating the need (and time) for patient enrollment. Examples of this are pharmacoeconomic analysis and meta-analysis. For example, we observed a patient who had a high serum digoxin level but who was asymptomatic from digoxin toxicity. We had previously published an analysis of a large data set quantifying the total costs of digoxin toxicity (Reference 7). In this analysis, most costs could be attributed to the time spent in the hospital (or the daily cost of an intensive care or regular ward bed). As our discussion of managing this patient ensued, the issue of giving digoxin immune Fab fragments arose. Administering it to the patient was rejected because this effective form of therapy is indicated only for "life-threatening" digoxin toxicity. But why? Couldn't we administer

digoxin immune Fab to save costs and discharge the patient more quickly? To answer this, we performed an economic analysis to balance the cost of digoxin immune Fab and the cost of the projected hospital stay. We found that it could indeed be cost-effective to administer this therapy to those with *non*-life-threatening digoxin toxicity, depending on the patient's renal function and digoxin plasma concentration at admission (Reference 8).

Meta-analysis is the statistical combination of similar small studies (already published) that, by themselves, may not be powered to detect differences in some outcomes (e.g., in mortality) to make a much more powerful study. We have performed several of these (References 9, 10). Again, performing an analysis and reanalysis of existing data or published studies can be an efficient form of scholarship for a Pharm.D. student that obviates the need for prospective patient recruitment and sometimes IRB approval. However, both examples given require research skills generally not conveyed to Pharm.D. students (e.g., expertise in decision analysis, sensitivity analysis). Therefore, choosing a mentor(s) with these talents is crucial; the learning experience can provide a good first step toward acquiring these skills and launching your research career as an independent investigator.

*In Vitro Studies*
My example of an in vitro intravenous stability study at the beginning of the chapter is appropriate. This form of research can be completely laboratory based. However, it does require the researcher to develop the specific laboratory skills necessary to complete the project (i.e., in this case, the ability to perform phenytoin assays and melting point determinations, which I learned from my faculty mentors). Other examples of this type of study can be performed rather efficiently. In another instance, we wanted to analyze the fate and significance of digitalis-like immunoreactive substance in renal transplant recipients (Reference 11). This study was performed prospectively—but the digoxin assays were performed as clinically indicated. In other words, no specific intervention such as a blood draw for the study was made; rather, existing blood was used to perform several assays. So, although this required IRB approval and consent, the methodology was relatively simple. Again, skills in assay performance and pharmacokinetic analysis were necessary. This idea arose from a Pharm.D. student when we were discussing problems with interpreting serum digoxin assays during his clerkship experience.

*Practice Evaluation Projects*

Clinical pharmacists are quite fond of studies that evaluate the impact of their clinical practice. We have grown accustomed to justifying our worth. Indeed, these evaluation projects can be valuable whether internally or shared broadly, and they can be used by others. For example, we had grown frustrated by patients who received chronic oral amiodarone being lost to follow-up and sometimes reappearing with severe adverse effects such as pulmonary toxicity. Therefore, we initiated a once-weekly collaborative "amiodarone clinic" (analogous to a warfarin clinic) based on the premise that these patients required scrutiny and follow-up, including laboratory monitoring and dosage adjustment. Later, we retrospectively evaluated the outcomes of this clinic compared with usual medical care (patients receiving amiodarone not being followed in our clinic) (Reference 12). This clinical care model has now been replicated relatively often, with Pharm.D. students integrated within the care team. Although this evaluation was performed at a single site, it had some impact because it was new and unique at the time. Be cautious of "quality assurance" or medication use evaluations as research projects. Let's say you want to discover the percentage of patients receiving amiodarone who are being followed appropriately and according to guidelines. Through the hospital database, a chart review is completed. But your findings are only for a single hospital and thus may not reflect care in the United States or even regionally. Therefore, although these data may be important for internal quality improvement purposes, they are often not publishable. The use of large, multicenter data sets would be more appropriate in this instance.

My intent in reviewing examples of small studies that you may consider is not to discourage you from experiences that are more ambitious. Rather, it is to suggest ways to efficiently gain some research experience during your Pharm.D. program. Your goals should be to develop skills in preparation for the residency program (and the required project) and to distinguish yourself in this respect, which should aid in your quest to secure a residency position. Occasionally, a Pharm.D. student will develop a relationship with a faculty member whereby he or she engages in research for a longer period, either as a paid or unpaid research assistant or through a series of research electives during a 2- to 3-year period. Moreover, some colleges (e.g., mine) have dual degree programs with the Pharm.D., such as a master's degree in clinical science, in which a clinical research project is required for completing the master's portion. These more intense research experiences will allow time to initiate and complete a more complex prospective clinical trial. Although some of the examples I suggested do not require IRB approval, I believe it is a great experience to go through this process and, again, something to add to your skill set that will aid in your performance during the residency. All IRBs require human subjects' training or education before the investigator can submit a proposal or participate in the research; this training, in and of itself, is quite valuable to a Pharm.D. student. Finally, most of the examples I have provided can be considered observational and "hypothesis-generating" research. You may have detected an association between two variables—but the next question should be *why*? And answering that question should be your *next* research project! In this way, you can develop a theme of research. Always be thinking about your next step and your next project in answering the research question(s). The results of research experiments answer some questions but always raise others.

### Complete the Research and Analyze the Data

Completing the research is the hard part (and the most time-consuming—be prepared to put in long hours), and analyzing the results is the fun part. Be prepared for pitfalls—research rarely proceeds as perfectly as planned. If you are using retrospective data that require chart review, design a comprehensive form to collect the patient data (after IRB approval, of course). Be extremely meticulous in your record keeping. If you plan to share your results through presentation or publication, they may be challenged. You have a responsibility for the accuracy and completeness of the data contained in the study. At the end of the day, your purpose is to help patients and their drug treatment with your research, and this work will carry your name. Although it is hoped otherwise, research findings and interpretations are occasionally later found to be incorrect; this should not be because of sloppy or dishonest record keeping or data analysis on the investigator's part. As a Pharm.D. student, you will most likely require the assistance of your mentor and possibly the assistance of outside experts (e.g., statisticians).

### Disseminate the Results

Here are the fruits of your labor. It's well and good to present your findings to your preceptor or to (for example) the Pharmacy and Therapeutics Committee (for a medication quality assurance project), but who else knows? At best, your findings will have some local impact. I encourage you not to stop at these internal venues—share them with the world! Consider the traditional steps that academic clinical faculty members would take in disseminating their findings.

## Write an Abstract for Submission to a Professional Meeting

Writing an abstract is a simple but acquired skill. Likely, your first attempt will be a miserable experience filled with the red lines and comments of your mentor. On reviewing my first abstract, the late Dr. Kenneth Rosen informed me that it was the very worst he had ever had the pleasure of reading. I got better at it, as will you. It's actually somewhat formulaic: one sentence to review the problem, one sentence about the purpose of the study or hypothesis, several sentences for methodology, several sentences for the results, one or two sentences for conclusions—and presto, you have an abstract. Use several abbreviations to save space, and if you want to get fancy and have room, try to insert a table or figure that shows key results. You must structure your abstract according to the guidelines of the professional society that hosts the meeting, so follow these guidelines carefully regarding format and word limit. Most abstracts are peer reviewed, and the acceptance rate will vary according to the professional society. Depending on the project, pharmacists and pharmacy students or residents are not limited to presenting their findings at pharmacy meetings; submitting them to various medical specialty meetings is open. However, getting an abstract accepted at the American College of Cardiology is much more difficult than, for example, at the American Society of Health-System Pharmacists midyear meeting. After submitting your abstract, you will receive notice whether it was accepted or not. If accepted, then what?

## Make a Platform or Poster Presentation

The abstract, if accepted, will generally be published, together with all the others in some format. Some are published in the official journal of the professional society (a real citation for your CV). But the purpose of submitting your abstract is to formally present your results at a (usually) national forum. This presentation may take two forms: an oral platform presentation or a poster session. Oral presentations are generally time-limited: 10–12 minutes for the presentation and 3 minutes for questions. The organization of a platform presentation should follow that of the abstract, and you will have only 10–12 minutes to share with everyone what has dominated your life for the past year. A rule of thumb is about 1 minute per slide, so two or three slides for background and purpose, two or three slides for methodology, two or three slides for results (with easy to read graphs and tables), and one or two slides for conclusions. Because of nerves and time constraints, I always recommend a typed script and insist on the student's or resident's simply reading the script for each slide. Remember, this is not a poetry recital; rather, it's a scientific session, so no one in the audience cares how eloquent you are—people in the audience are just interested in the findings. The worst presentations are those that ramble on and go over the allotted time limit. Remember to make the slides easy to read and follow. The moderator has the responsibility and authority to yank you, if need be. In addition, practice makes perfect: you should practice in a formal way several times to a variety of audiences so that you can field potential questions and make sure of your timing before the actual presentation. Fortunately (for you, anyway), most professional groups are now emphasizing poster presentations rather than platform presentations. Here, you prepare a poster for display (in a large room filled with others), and attendees peruse the session viewing the posters. They may (or may not) stop to ask you questions about your work. It's certainly a more leisurely and less stressful way to present your research. Occasionally, you may be challenged – but at least 1,000 people aren't watching you get hammered. Also, professional networking is much more likely to occur. Again, the poster should be organized according to the abstract; you will have room for complementary figures, tables, and references (Figure 3).

## Write the Paper for Submission to a Journal

This is the proof of the pudding—though many fail to take this last important step (Figure 4). In my view, writing scientific papers, like writing abstracts, is an acquired skill, and your first attempt will more than likely be a frustrating experience. The first draft with its impressive quantities of red ink from your mentor should be kept as a fond memory that you can reflect on years down the road. If your mentor is an experienced scientist, it will take many such ugly drafts. Your mentor may also make changes to his or her own changes. You should have an idea which journal you are contemplating before submitting a final version of the manuscript because each one may have a slightly different required format. Read the "Instructions for Authors" page in the specific journal very carefully. The specific journal to choose requires some thought. Is your study aimed mainly at pharmacists, or would it be valuable to a broader range of health professionals? Some journals are much more discerning in their criteria for acceptance (i.e., it's much more difficult to get your paper accepted for publication). In general, journals with a high impact factor (IF) are more prestigious and more difficult. In clinical medicine, the *New England Journal of Medicine* has one of the highest IFs (about 35); you can view others to get a sense of relative difficulty. Each journal generally lists its IF on its Web site. In general, I usually recommend that

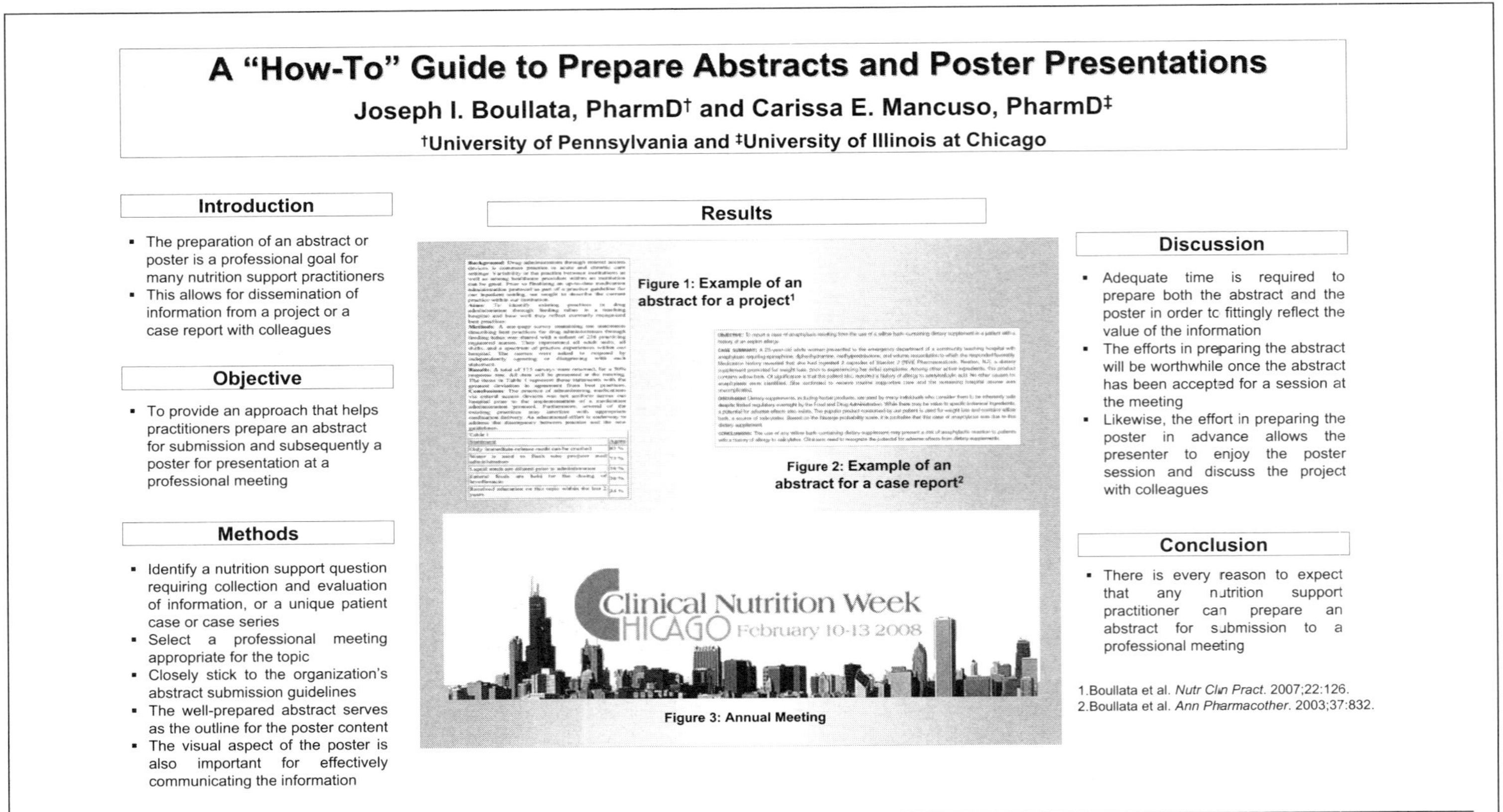

**Figure 3.** Example of a scientific poster.
Reprinted with permission from Sage Publications. Boullata JI, Mancuso CE. A "how-to" guide in preparing abstracts and poster presentations. Nutr Clin Pract 2007;22:641-6.

your first attempt be to a journal with the highest degree of prestige and readership with a reasonable chance at acceptance. The paper may be rejected or not even reviewed, but seasoned scholars have become accustomed to such failures. When submitting your paper to be considered for publication (unless it is rejected outright), you will receive a review or critique of it. It may be rejected because of this review, but sometimes, the review is quite helpful in your planned submission to a different journal. Alternatively, you may receive an invitation to revise the manuscript on the basis of the reviewers' comments. Take the invitation to revise and address each of the reviewer's points carefully (and politely); then, submit a revised version. Seldom will a paper be accepted without some form of revision. Afterward, you will receive a letter (or likely an e-mail) that your revised paper has been accepted for publication. At this time, and only at this time, you may break out the champagne. Thereafter, you will receive a "galley proof" of your paper to approve or see what it will look like in the journal when published. Go through this carefully, and ask others to review these galleys. More than once, I have been embarrassed at typos or errors that I missed in the galleys. Although you have completed a major accomplishment and taken a clinical problem from the idea stage to research to publication, your responsibility does not cease. Now, a paper is there with your results for all to see (and discern) with your name on it. You and your coauthors are responsible to the scientific community for its contents and findings.

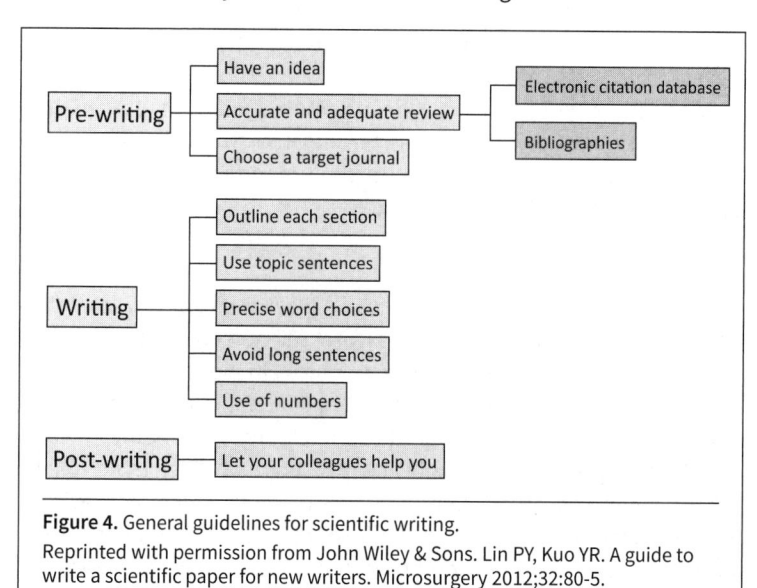

**Figure 4.** General guidelines for scientific writing.
Reprinted with permission from John Wiley & Sons. Lin PY, Kuo YR. A guide to write a scientific paper for new writers. Microsurgery 2012;32:80-5.

## Other Forms of Scholarly Contributions for Pharm.D. Students
In this chapter, I have concentrated on the completion of the small research projects a Pharm.D. student may contemplate. However, other forms of scholarly contributions can be considered, and completion of these can also be a highly valued experience that distinguishes you from other residency candidates. The two examples I will use are case reports and review papers.

### Case Reports
During your experiential training, you will observe and help care for interesting patients; one or two of them may present unique problems or questions related to their drug therapy. Examples may be an unusual and infrequently reported adverse event or a surprising and novel response to a drug therapy. Your first step in writing this patient case for publication is to complete a thorough literature search. You may find the report of the adverse event not as uncommon as you first thought. If so and if the patient you observed will add little to the current literature, then abandon your efforts. If, however, you decide in conversations with your preceptor that value may exist in the case for others, then proceed. Although some IRBs do not require approval for a case report, I think it is wise to seek it.

Although once common, many journals no longer accept case reports. For the journals that do still accept case reports, read the instructions for authors carefully, and review examples of previously published case reports for format and style. Proving cause and effect is generally the Achilles' heel of getting case reports published; yet there are published methods to assist in making this determination (Reference 13). I always urge potential authors of case reports to seriously contemplate the value and strength of the anticipated case report.

### Review Papers
Papers reviewing the drug treatment of a disease or the characteristics of a new drug are highly valued by practitioners and often cited by scientific authors. If these papers are done well, they are quite difficult to write and very time-consuming. When contemplating such a paper, again perform a complete literature search and ask whether this review will bring value to the audience. Has it already been done well by others? When I am going over papers for publication that are reviews, several common features annoy me (and subsequently, I render a harsh review). First, there are reviews that simply regurgitate the findings of published studies paragraph after paragraph (e.g., "this study designed

as such showed this, and that study designed this way showed that, blah, blah, blah"). Valuable reviews are those written by experts who can synthesize others' findings and put them into perspective; they may interject their own opinions, which, as the opinions of experts, I value. Pharm.D. students, by definition, are not yet experts. Second, there are reviews that overly criticize published studies (as Pharm.D. students are taught to do in Drug Information class). For instance: "This study (published as the lead article in the *New England Journal of Medicine*) failed to do this or consider that." If you are the world's expert on this area and have completed major studies in the area, you can criticize, but if you aren't and haven't, you can't. Nonetheless, the act of compiling (and reading) the entire literature on a subject should be quite valuable for a Pharm.D. student. It could provide ideas and fodder for future projects.

> As a pharmacy student, I wish I had been involved in some type of research project to help me prepare for tackling a resident research project.
>
> —Joshua Elder, 2011/12 PGY2 Pediatrics Resident at Riley Hospital for Children at Indiana University Health, Indianapolis, Ind.

## CONCLUSION

In summary, I highly encourage Pharm.D. students to actively seek research experience during their Pharm.D. education, particularly if they plan to complete a PGY1 residency (and beyond). Research and scholarly projects can be highly rewarding, can add to your skill set, and may have impactful findings that help patient care. They can also lead to career-long relationships with faculty mentors and collaborators. Applied research experience can also increase your competitiveness in getting accepted into the residency of your choice. And who knows—your first experience may cause you to pursue clinical research as a career and eventually become a dean.

## ACKNOWLEDGMENT

*I would like to thank Larisa Cavallari, Pharm.D., FCCP, BCPS, for her helpful comments in preparing this chapter.*

## REFERENCES

1. Bauman JL, Siepler JK. Intravenous phenytoin (concluded). N Engl J Med 1976;296:111.
2. Bauman JL, Siepler JK, Fitzloff J. Phenytoin crystallization in intravenous fluids. Drug Intell Clin Pharm 1977;11:646-9.
3. Kim SE, Whittington JI, Nguyen LM, Ambrose PJ, Corelli RL. Pharmacy students' perceptions of a required senior research project. Am J Pharm Educ 2010;74:1-7.
4. Boyer EL. A Special Report. Scholarship Reconsidered. Priorities of the Professoriate. The Carnegie Foundation for the Advancement of Teaching, 1990.
5. Barbarash RA, Bauman JL, Lukazewski AA, Srebro JP, Rich S. Verapamil infusions in the treatment of atrial tachyarrhythmias. Crit Care Med 1986;14:886-8.
6. Oberg KC, O'Toole MF, Gallastegui JL, Bauman JL. Observations in patients with "late" proarrhythmia due to quinidine. Am J Cardiol 1994;74:192-4.
7. Ghandi A, Vlasses PH, Morton D, Bauman JL. Economic impact of digoxin toxicity. Pharmacoeconomics 1997;12:175-81.
8. DiDomenico R, Sanoski CA, Walton SM, Bauman JL. Analysis of the use of digoxin immune Fab for the treatment of non-life-threatening digoxin toxicity. J Cardiovasc Pharmacol Ther 2000;5:77-85.
9. Roberts SA, Viana M, Nazari J, Bauman JL. Invasive and noninvasive methods to determine the effectiveness of amiodarone in sustained ventricular tachycardia. A compilation of clinical observations using meta-analysis. Pace Clin Electrophysiol 1994;17:1590-602.
10. Southworth MR, Viana M, Bauman JL. A comparison of quinidine and sotalol for the maintenance of normal sinus rhythm in patients with chronic atrial fibrillation. Am J Cardiol 1999;83:1629-32.
11. Schrader BJ, Maddux MS, Veremis SA, Moses MR, Maturen A, Bauman JL. Digitalis-like-immunoreactive substance in renal transplant recipients. J Clin Pharmacol 1991;31:1126-31.
12. Sanoski C, Schoen MD, Gonzalez RC, Avital B, Bauman JL. Rationale, development and outcomes of a multidisciplinary clinic for patients receiving chronic oral amiodarone. Pharmacotherapy 1998;18:146S-151S.
13. Naranjo CA, Busto U, Sellers EM, et al. A method for estimating the probability of adverse drug reactions. Clin Pharmacol Ther 1981;30:239-45.

## OTHER SUGGESTED READING

1. Alexandrov AV, Hennerici MG. Writing good abstracts. Cerebrovasc Dis 2007;23:256-9.
2. Boullata JI, Mancuso CE. A "how-to" guide in preparing abstracts and poster presentations. Nutr Clin Pract 2007;22:641-6.
3. Chernick V. How to get your paper accepted for publication. Paediatr Respir Rev 2012;13:130-2.

4. Cohen H. How to write a patient case report. Am J Health Syst Pharm 2006;63:1888-92.
5. Lashford LS. Presenting a scientific paper, including the pitfalls. Arch Dis Child 1995;73:168-9.
6. Lin PY, Kuo YR. A guide to write a scientific paper for new writers. Microsurgery 2012;32:80-5.

# STEP IX
# DOCUMENT IT ALL

Garrett E. Schramm, Pharm.D., BCPS
Heather A. Personett, Pharm.D., BCPS
Erin M. Nystrom, Pharm.D., BCNSP

## ABBREVIATIONS IN THIS CHAPTER

| | |
|---|---|
| APPE | Advanced pharmacy practice experience |
| CV | Curriculum vitae |
| IPPE | Introductory pharmacy practice experience |
| PGY1 | Postgraduate year one |
| PGY2 | Postgraduate year two |
| RAP | Residency application portfolio |
| RPD | Residency program director |

The goal of the *ACCP Field Guide to Becoming a Standout Pharmacy Residency Candidate* Step IX: Document It All chapter is to provide tips and tools to help students market their skills and experience effectively through curriculum vitae writing and portfolio development.

## INTRODUCTION

Compared with their predecessors, pharmacy students have never been better prepared to enter the workforce. The combination of outstanding critical thinking skills with technological advances, state-of-the-art teaching facilities, and valuable work experience has created a residency candidate who can succeed in a plethora of pharmacy settings. Moreover, the pursuit of postgraduate residency training has led to countless opportunities that can further differentiate resident candidate's career paths from that of their peers. However, given the appeal of residency training, an unfortunate disparity exists between the number of qualified applicants and the number of available postgraduate positions. According to the 2012 National Matching Service results, 3,706 postgraduate year one (PGY1) applicants participated in the Resident Matching Program (Reference 1). Of those students, 1,438 (38.8%) failed to match with a PGY1 residency program. Although these results may be discouraging, they suggest that the ability of applicants to "sell" themselves in such a competitive environment has never been more important. A well-designed curriculum vitae (CV) is a powerful tool used by residency program applicants to communicate their experience and accomplishments and thus elevate themselves above their peers.

A CV is a biographical synopsis of one's professional experience and accomplishments organized in an easy-to-read format for prospective employers to quickly assess applicants for the position they are looking to fill. The Latin origin of the term *curriculum vitae* translates into "the course of one's life" and differs from a one- or two-page resume, which typically focuses on one's educational background, work experience, and pertinent skills related to the available position. A CV is considered by many a more elaborate "academic resume" used by individuals in the pharmacy profession who are seeking positions in academia, research, postgraduate training, and management. Unlike a resume, a CV offers the ability to provide a more detailed description of your experiences, such that the employer gains additional insight on your education, training, work experience, research, and other notable accomplishments. The length of a CV depends on how thoroughly you expand on the details related to the individual experiences listed in your CV.

Securing a desired position is often influenced by effectively communicating the experiences and accomplishments highlighted in your CV. For many pharmacy students, the pressure associated with developing a CV can be a potential source of confusion and anxiety. As you build this document, you will soon realize that this dynamic record is as unique as you are. This chapter is designed to provide tips and tools to help you successfully market your skills and experiences through CV writing.

## ESTABLISHING A SENSE OF ACCOMPLISHED CONFIDENCE
### Emotional Introspection
The initial developmental stages of a CV can introduce a mixture of emotions. Reflecting on your accomplishments may well lead to a heightened sense of pride, especially with the notation of your newly acquired skills. Alternatively, some may fear that this type of documentation will be perceived as pretentious. The pressure of obtaining a residency may further amplify these emotional highs and lows. Before constructing a CV, you may consider applying emotional introspection,

the act of looking within oneself, to establish and maintain a sense of accomplished confidence. This should not be confused with arrogance; rather, it is a form of self-assurance gained through life experience, an appropriate balance of pride and humility. Preparing a CV by first applying emotional introspection will lead to the development of a confident individual with a competitive CV to match. Self-reflection with subsequent documentation of relevant educational experiences and accomplishments will augment a sense of pride in your body of work. This will make the process more enjoyable and fulfilling as you begin telling the story of your professional life.

### Directed Message

The fundamental purpose of a CV is to effectively communicate how your experience and accomplishments are relevant to the available position. Doing so in a descriptive, yet succinct manner is of paramount importance because a residency program director (RPD) will likely have limited time to review large volumes of CVs for a set number of positions. The goal of RPDs is straightforward: to find the best candidate for their program by assessing various criteria. Although a uniform consensus of desirable resident qualities is not available, RPDs usually review a CV looking for evidence of pharmacotherapeutic knowledge, clinical training exposure as demonstrated through introductory and advanced pharmacy practice experiences (IPPEs, APPEs), research experience, leadership roles, involvement in the community and pharmacy profession, and other outcomes or awards. Through the content in your CV, you face the challenge of highlighting accomplishments in the aforementioned areas to show that the training and skills obtained in pharmacy school will be a positive addition to a residency program. The following discussion will provide general considerations for clearly displaying the message you wish to convey.

## IDENTIFYING THE TARGET AUDIENCE

After your period of self-reflection and development of a directed message, it is important to consider researching your program(s) of interest to determine how to individualize your CV content. Residency Web sites often provide insight on the purpose of the program, resident goals and objectives, required core rotations, longitudinal experiences, and faculty members. This creates an opportunity to customize your CV to appeal to the RPD and clinical faculty by highlighting the skills and accomplishments you hold that are consistent with the purpose of a particular program.

Students often assume that once a CV is submitted for consideration, the RPD is the only individual who reviews it. This may be true; however, in some situations, the RPD may elect to form a selection panel to evaluate applications before extending interview offers. The makeup of such a selection panel may include current pharmacy residents, other RPDs, assistant RPDs, preceptors, and human resources representatives. To gain a competitive advantage, you are encouraged to ask the RPD whether the applications and accompanying CVs are reviewed only by the RPD or by several individuals and then tailor your CVs accordingly. For example, if you learn that the postgraduate year two (PGY2) RPD in nutrition support pharmacy will be reviewing PGY1 applications and find this specialty particularly appealing, highlighting your interest or experiences related to this specialty may be beneficial. Alternatively, if you are undecided about your plans (i.e., PGY2 specialty training), you are encouraged to develop a well-rounded CV that does not exclude any particular specialty. Regardless of your plans, the more details you know about the selection process, the better equipped you will be to emphasize pertinent experiences and accomplishments.

> *I wish I had updated my CV monthly or every other month. I found it difficult to remember all of the extracurricular activities I participated in when I only updated my CV yearly.*
>
> —Jennifer Grelle, 2011/12 PGY1 Pharmacotherapy Specialty Resident at Texas Tech Health Sciences Center School of Pharmacy, Amarillo, Tex.

## QUALITIES OF A DESIRABLE CV

You will soon discover that a recipe for the "perfect" CV does not exist. Content and formatting are largely scripted from individual preferences, prior examples, and all manner of feedback. The afforded freedom to define what qualities comprise a desirable CV can be equally refreshing and frustrating. A CV may be the story of your life; yet, to have the desired effect, the content must be periodically (e.g., quarterly) updated to display your continued growth in a fashion that is easily navigated and understood by others. Despite the lack of universally accepted elements, formatting, and related content, the generally accepted qualities of a desirable CV are outlined in Table 1. These qualities are minimum expectations in the assessment of an individual's candidacy.

Rather than focus solely on what information should be included in a CV, equal attention should be dedicated to avoiding certain errors. Indeed, your candidacy may be compromised by typographic, grammatical, and spelling mistakes, which the RPD or selection panel typically views as inattention to detail. Unusual font size and type, use of graphics, and

Table 1. General Qualities of a Desirable CV

| Quality | Comment(s) |
|---|---|
| Avoidance of typographic mistakes | Compliance with correct spelling and grammar is expected of pharmacy professionals. |
| Easy-to-follow format and organization | A CV should follow an easily understood format and logical organization to reduce confusion by the reviewer. If elaborate listings are required under a single heading, consider incorporating subheadings (i.e., presentations may be subcategorized as Local, Regional, State, or National). |
| Easy to read | Appropriate font size and type allow the reviewer to quickly assess content. Expanding on details should be done in a bulleted rather than paragraph format to aid in timely assessment. |
| Relevant content | Irrelevant details decrease the quality of the content. Consider listing only information that pertains to the position to which you are applying. Past degrees and unique awards or roles before pharmacy school are appropriate. |
| Reversed chronologic order | Listing the most recent facts, followed by older facts or descriptors, allows the reviewer to quickly assess the progression of your skills or training. |
| Succinct descriptions, elaborations, or explanations | Targeted content without superfluous information allows the reviewer to quickly assess the candidate. Action verbs are recommended to describe a particular skill or experience. |

unplanned formatting issues because of differences in word processing software, although easily overlooked by the CV's author, may have disastrous consequences when assessed by those in the selection process.

## LISTING AND ORGANIZING CONTENT

The layout and content of a CV is ultimately up to the individual. You must consider how you will organize the content to best represent your candidacy for the position. You will undoubtedly have examples to aid in developing a CV; however, the goal is to create an individualized document that distinguishes your qualifications from those of another candidate. After constructing a list of relevant skills, experiences, and training opportunities, you will need to develop an outline with individual headings to organize the information. Box 1 lists CV headings that may be considered when developing your document. Once you have organized all the information under the selected headings, you should consider the content outline. The following content is based on the authors' recommendations and is not an exhaustive template. Appendix 1 provides a sample CV for your reference. You are encouraged to consider including a header or footer on your CV that outlines your name and chronologic page number to ease navigation for the reviewer(s).

## Personal Information

The purpose of providing personal information on a CV is twofold: first, to identify the candidate, and second, to provide contact information. The amount of professional information provided is up to you; however, a legal name, current address, and contact information (telephone number(s) and e-mail address) is sufficient to fulfill this purpose. It is imperative that accurate and current information be included in this section to ensure that contact can be established if a residency interview is extended. Professional judgment on the appropriateness of the e-mail address and voicemail greeting is expected. Once contact (e.g., electronic or verbal) is established, you are highly encouraged to use

---

**Box 1.** Possible curriculum vitae headings.

- Academic and Professional Presentations
- Administration and Leadership Experience
- Advanced Pharmacy Practice Experience
- Community or Volunteer Service
- Education
- Honors and Awards
- Introductory Pharmacy Practice Experience
- Personal/Contact Information
- Professional Certification
- Professional Experience
- Professional Licensure
- Professional Meeting Attendance
- Professional Memberships and Activities
- Publications
- Research Experience
- Teaching Experience

professional communication practices at all times and avoid informal responses. Additional details including age, sex, ethnicity, religious beliefs, marital status, and photographs are unnecessary to assess one's candidacy for the available position.

Example CVs may include "Curriculum Vitae" or "CV" in the heading of personal information. Although the merit of adding this terminology is arguable, most residency programs specifically request a CV, thereby negating the need to state the obvious.

## Education

After personal information, a reverse chronology of education is typically listed on the CV. Rather than listing a school first, it is suggested that you list your degree(s), followed by the institution, location, and expected or conferred graduation date(s). Education that did not lead to a degree (e.g., general studies or pre-pharmacy) may be considered for inclusion if you deem the experience relevant to your career trajectory. Including your GPA may be appropriate if the residency program does not ask for transcripts with the application packet. Any graduation honors (e.g., *cum laude, magna cum laude*, or *summa cum laude*) indicate academic distinction and would be excellent additions to this particular heading.

## Licensure and Certifications

Most students acquire internship licensure during pharmacy school as a requirement to participate in IPPEs or APPEs. Disclosing all licensure information is necessary if potential employers conduct a thorough background check. The license state of origin and registration number should be included in the CV to verify that your licensure is in good standing. Updates of active or inactive status are expected.

Attainment of certifications (e.g., Basic Life Support, Advanced Cardiac Life Support) symbolizes professional development and may be required for particular program enrollments. Other certifications (e.g., immunization delivery) inform the reviewer of unique skill sets or training. What constitutes relevant pharmacy licenses and certifications is ultimately at your discretion; however, guidance from a professional mentor, professor, or preceptor is recommended.

## Employment and Professional Experience

Selection panels and RPDs may assess employment and professional experiences to determine your degree of exposure to a particular area(s) of interest. For many students, IPPEs and APPEs are assigned; however, a short description of your responsibilities for employment and professional experiences shows their relevance to residency training. To avoid expansive descriptions in paragraph format, bullet points beginning with suggested action verbs (Table 2) may be used to delineate individual experiences. For content length, be descriptive yet concise. Use at least two bullet points, but no more than five. Use of descriptions that are more extensive can be onerous to the reviewer.

### Presentations, Research, and Publications

Public speaking is an integral component of residency training and your future role as a clinical pharmacist. Documenting your public speaking experience will provide insight into your possible areas of interest, ability to speak to a vast array of audience members, and continual refinement of speaking skills. With respect to presentation listing, the format may vary; however, the title of the presentation, date, venue, and description of the audience will provide adequate information for assessment. Informal discussions (e.g., patient reviews, group work, team-building exercises) that are part of everyday training should not be included under the Presentation heading.

Before or during pharmacy school, you may capitalize on research opportunities to gain additional exposure before residency training. You may find that previous experience eases the transition from student to resident; however, many students enter PGY1 residencies without formal research training. If you are fortunate enough to contribute to research, the evidence for it should be clearly outlined. The content under the Research Experience heading may include the title of the project, location, name of advisor(s) with appropriate credentials, and descriptors of your role. If the research resulted in a publication, a separate heading of Publication(s) is recommended. The research publication should be referenced in the style adopted by the National Library of Medicine, and journal titles should conform to those used in the *Index Medicus* (Reference 2).

Publications of book chapters, reviews, or online work should be included as well. Local or institutional publications that are not discoverable (e.g., Pharmacy and Therapeutics monographs, medication reviews, hospital newsletters) may be listed with a short description of your role. If a heading lacks listed experiences or perhaps lends itself to another established area, you should strongly consider excluding this section or seek professional mentoring advice for suggested placement. Of note, you should be prepared to discuss all content in your CV and to provide expanded details to a potential employer upon request.

**Table 2.** Action Verbs Used to Describe Employment and Professional Experiences

| Management or Technical Skills | Communication or Teaching Skills | Research or Creative Skills |
|---|---|---|
| • Administered | • Addressed | • Clarified |
| • Assembled | • Advised | • Collected |
| • Assigned | • Arranged | • Conceptualized |
| • Attained | • Clarified | • Created |
| • Chaired | • Corresponded | • Critiqued |
| • Clarified | • Coached | • Developed |
| • Coordinated | • Coordinated | • Directed |
| • Developed | • Developed | • Established |
| • Directed | • Drafted | • Evaluated |
| • Enabled | • Edited | • Examined |
| • Encouraged | • Enlisted | • Extracted |
| • Evaluated | • Evaluated | • Identified |
| • Increased | • Explained | • Inspected |
| • Maintained | • Formulated | • Integrated |
| • Organized | • Influenced | • Interpreted |
| • Planned | • Interpreted | • Interviewed |
| • Prioritized | • Lectured | • Invented |
| • Recommended | • Moderated | • Investigated |
| • Reviewed | • Negotiated | • Organized |
| • Scheduled | • Persuaded | • Performed |
| • Strengthened | • Publicized | • Planned |
| • Supervised | • Recruited | • Reviewed |
| • Trained | • Wrote | |

## HONORS AND AWARDS

As you progress through pharmacy school, you will attain honors and awards for individual or team efforts. Informational details of honors or awards should be outlined (i.e., name of honor or award and date received) to provide a clear description and understanding for review. Explanatory details should be included if the honor or award has unique selection criteria or if they might aid in the audience's understanding of relevance. Achievements attained before pharmacy school may be included if you feel the addition will be of great influence with the prospective employer. Ensure that any honors or awards contain appropriate facts and timescales rather than vague descriptors.

### Professional Organizations and Activities

Your involvement in professional organizations signifies a commitment to the pharmacy profession and invites opportunities for further development or refinement of leadership skills. Active participation in professional societies (i.e., local, regional, state, and national) is often encouraged or required of many pharmacy residents. Leadership roles highlighted on your CV may provide an RPD and selection panel with evidence of skills in communication, team building, and problem solving. You are encouraged to include short descriptions of your activities/role for each professional organization listed; however, in some situations, membership may be all that applies.

### Volunteer and Community Service

Volunteer and community service is a notable addition to any CV. The lessons learned through this experience will increase your understanding of the service component to patients and their families and will signify your ongoing development of leadership and organizational skills. Your documentation of community service activities should include the organization's name, timescale, and any necessary descriptors of your role. Particular attention to leadership opportunities within the community or volunteer services is an excellent opportunity for expansion.

## ELEMENTS TO AVOID

The importance of what to include in your CV should not be overshadowed by the equally fundamental concept of what not to include. Once you have completed a draft version, enlist the help of proofreaders to identify typographic mistakes and review the content. Enlisting the help of several proofreaders (e.g., faculty, mentors, employers) will increase the likelihood of finding errors and invite constructive feedback for continuous improvement.

Particular focus on the consistency of the CV's organization, capitalization, bulleting, and margin setup will lend the CV a professional appearance. Unorganized or inconsistent formatting will lead to difficulty in locating details, with possible inadvertent oversight of such details by the reviewer. If electronic means are used for CV submission, conversion to a Portable Document Format (PDF) will decrease the likelihood of formatting errors that can result from differences in application software.

Attention to detail includes determining whether the font size is too large or too small. In most situations, Times New Roman or Arial Narrow with 10- to 12-point fonts is appropriate, with bold or italics used sparingly to highlight key elements. Other unusual font styles should be avoided because of difficulty reading. An attempt to lengthen a CV by increasing font size or setting inconsistent margins is not advised. Suggested margins are defaulted on most word processing applications, which should facilitate printing on 8.5 × 11-inch paper while maintaining legibility and logical page breaks. Additional CV practices that should be avoided include using scented paper, using unprofessional paper color, using unexplained abbreviations, and including any artwork.

Finally, the content of the CV must remain factual at all times, especially in the setting of discoverable content on the Internet. If that information is viewed as discrepant, credibility may be compromised. Although many CVs may resemble one another, plagiarism is unacceptable.

## DEVELOPING AND MAINTAINING A PORTFOLIO

In addition to using a CV to document your achievements, consider developing a residency application portfolio (RAP) to track and reflect on your efforts within and outside pharmacy school in preparation for residency applications and interviews. Compared with a student portfolio, which is required of all pharmacy students by the Accreditation Council for Pharmacy Education, the RAP, in electronic or hard copy form, is a much more selective collection of academic achievements and practice experiences, chosen for inclusion on the basis of their relevancy to securing a residency position. The RAP's content encompasses that which is included in your CV and additional expanded highlights. For example, your RAP may include a table of contents, personal statement, CV, certificates, honors and awards, supporting documents for projects and presentations, scholarly activity, leadership examples, and performance assessments. These additions may provide further insight for an RPD and selection panel assessing your candidacy for a particular residency program.

You may not be asked to submit a RAP for a residency application or present it in an interview; however, the preparatory value is multifaceted. Developing and reviewing a RAP provide an excellent opportunity to reflect on accomplishments as you develop or update a CV, submit an application, and, in particular, prepare for a residency interview. As you formulate and later peruse your RAP, think about why a particular item was included, how it was used, and what was learned from the experience. As a residency candidate, you are expected to be intimately familiar with and to expand on your CV's content during an interview. A

RAP is an excellent means to ensure this happens. For example, when an interviewer asks for additional details related to a group project conducted during your first year of pharmacy school, developing a RAP will not only allow you to answer this question, but also may provide additional follow-up answers to questions related to the group's dynamics and overall success of the project.

Although the RAP may not be a necessary component of the residency application process, it can be a valuable tool to prepare for an interview, facilitate self-reflection, spark mental preparation, and instill confidence, all of which will help you stand out among your peers.

## CONCLUSION

The process of developing a CV can be an intimidating and overwhelming experience. Performing an emotional introspection and developing a targeted message before organizing your CV may simplify the process and increase pride in your achievements while documenting your experiences and accomplishments. An organized CV with succinct descriptions will allow RPDs and selection panels to quickly assess your candidacy. Developing a RAP will further augment your residency interview preparation. Careful consideration, preparation, and utilization of the tips and tools outlined in this chapter will help you market your skills and experience effectively through CV writing and RAP development.

## REFERENCES

1. ASHP Resident Matching Program for Positions Beginning in 2013 [homepage on the Internet]. Match Statistics. Statistics for Previous Years' Matches. Toronto, Ontario, Canada: National Matching Services. Available at www.natmatch.com/ashprmp/. Accessed September 2, 2012.
2. U.S. National Library of Medicine [homepage on the internet]. Bethesda, MD: National Institutes of Health. Available at www.nlm.nih.gov. Accessed September 2, 2012.

## SUGGESTED RESOURCE

1. American College of Clinical Pharmacy [homepage on the Internet]. Lenexa, KS: CV Preparation Tips: ACCP Online Curriculum Vitae Review Program. Available at www.accp.com/stunet/cv.aspx. Accessed August 28, 2012.

# APPENDIX 1. SAMPLE CV

## Sally A. Student
11068 Oak Spur Court, Apt G
Gator, Minnesota
(555) 555-1212 (home); (555) 555-2121 (cell)
sastudent@mycollegeofpharmacy.edu

### EDUCATION

**Doctor of Pharmacy Candidate**　　　　　　　　2008 – present
My College of Pharmacy
Big Town, Minnesota

**Bachelor of Science in Chemistry**　　　　　　　2004–2008
*Magna cum laude*
University of the Lakes
Small Town, Minnesota

### LICENSURE AND CERTIFICATIONS

**Pharmacy Intern License #000-000**　　　　　　2008 – present
Minnesota Board of Pharmacy

**Immunization Delivery Provider**　　　　　　　　2008 – present
American Pharmacists Association

**Basic Cardiac Life Support Provider**　　　　　　2008 – present
American Heart Association

### EMPLOYMENT EXPERIENCE

**Pharmacy Intern**　　　　　　　　　　　　　　　2009–2011
ABC Pharmacy Outlet
Hot Desert, Arizona
- Conducted adverse drug reaction reporting
- Filled automated dispensing devices (Pyxis)
- Filled and/or compounded prescription orders
- Delivered prescription orders to the proper hospital unit
- Packaged bulk medications into unit dose

**Chemistry Research Assistant**　　　　　　　　　2006–2008
University of the Lakes
Small Town, Minnesota
- Assisted in physical chemistry research under faculty advisement
- Prepared and delivered oral presentation for faculty
- Participated in statewide undergraduate research poster presentation
- Cowrote research update section of the Chemistry Department's monthly newsletter

## PROFESSIONAL EXPERIENCE

*Advanced Pharmacy Practice Experiences:*

**Community Pharmacy** — Pending
Gopher Pharmacy, Lake, Minnesota
Preceptor: Don Gopher, Pharm.D.

**Pediatrics** — Pending
Children's Clinic and Hospital, St. Louis, Missouri
Preceptor: Jenny Johnson, Pharm.D., BCPS

**Critical Care** — Pending
County Medical Center, Minneapolis, Minnesota
Preceptor: Bill Intensive, Pharm.D., FCCP, BCPS

**Internal Medicine II** — Pending
Academic Center, LaCrosse, Wisconsin
Preceptor: Jacob Johnson, Pharm.D.

**Cardiology** — November 2012
Heart and Lung Hospital, Sioux Falls, South Dakota
Preceptor: Rhythm Torsades, Pharm.D., BCPS

**Infectious Diseases** — October 2012
Community Hospital and Clinics, Des Moines, Iowa
Preceptor: John Smith, Pharm.D., BCPS (AQ-ID)

**Ambulatory Care – Geriatrics** — September 2012
Wally Drug and Card Shop, Great Lake, Minnesota
Preceptor: Joseph Smith, Pharm.D.

**Ambulatory Care – Psychiatry** — August 2012
State Hospital, Big Hill, South Dakota
Preceptor: Susie Johnson, Pharm.D., BCPP

**Internal Medicine I** — July 2012
Big Academic Center, Rochester, Minnesota
Preceptor: Timothy Johnson, Pharm.D., FCCP, BCPS

**Hospital Pharmacy Practice** — May – June 2012
University of Mayo, Rochester, Minnesota
Preceptor: Paul Smith, R.Ph.

*Introductory Pharmacy Practice Experiences:*

**Community IPPE** — May 2011
Wally Drug and Card Shop, Great Lake, Minnesota
Preceptor: Joseph Smith, Pharm.D.

**Institutional IPPE** — June 2011
University of Mayo, Rochester, Minnesota
Preceptor: Paul Smith, R.Ph.

## RESEARCH EXPERIENCE

**"Assessment of Student Workload on Quality of Life Parameters"**     2012–2013
My College of Pharmacy
Big Town, Minnesota
- Pharmacy Student Project
- Co-designed, administered, and analyzed a survey-based assessment of 150 first-year pharmacy students
- Determined positive and negative predictors of workload balance

Advisers: Heather Personett, Pharm.D., BCPS; Erin Nystrom, Pharm.D., BCNSP

**"Analysis of Ligand-to-Metal Charge Transfer of Europium"**     2006–2008
University of the Lakes
Small Town, Minnesota
- Chemistry Research Assistant Project
- Prepared samples for quantitative assessment
- Conducted assessment of energy charge transfer
- Analyzed results and co-wrote manuscript for planned submission
- Presented research at statewide undergraduate poster presentation

Adviser: John Johnson, Ph.D.

## PRESENTATIONS

### *Student Presentations:*

**"An Overview of Diabetes"**     January 2013
Big Academic Center, Rochester, Minnesota
Pharmacy Education Specialty Day
Audience: Clinical Pharmacist Faculty and Residents

**"USP 797 Review"**     November 2012
University of Mayo, Rochester, Minnesota
Central Pharmacist Education Hour
Audience: Staff Pharmacists and Technicians

## COMMITTEE WORK

**Dean's Advisory Panel**     2011–2012
My College of Pharmacy
Big Town, Minnesota

**Pharmacy School Social Committee**     2011–2012
My College of Pharmacy
Big Town, Minnesota

**Big Brother Big Sister Planning Committee**     2008–2010
My Hometown, Minnesota

| **PROFESSIONAL ORGANIZATIONS AND ACTIVITIES** | |
|---|---|
| American Society of Health-System Pharmacists Student | 2011 – present |
| American College of Clinical Pharmacy Student | 2010 – present |
| My State's Society of Health-System Pharmacists | 2008 – present |

| **HONORS AND AWARDS** | |
|---|---|
| **Rho Chi Honor Society**<br>• Member | 2008 – present |
| **Outstanding First-Year Pharmacy Student Award**<br>• Awarded to top student in first-year pharmacy class | 2008 |
| **Some Name Memorial Achievement Award**<br>• A merit-based scholarship presented to pharmacy students who display excellence in teamwork with other professions | 2009 |

# STEP X

# STEP UP TO THE PLATE: BRINGING IT HOME IN YOUR FINAL PROFESSIONAL YEAR

Beth Bryles Phillips, Pharm.D., FCCP, BCPS

## ABBREVIATIONS IN THIS CHAPTER

| | |
|---|---|
| ACCP | American College of Clinical Pharmacy |
| APPE | Advanced pharmacy practice experience |
| ASHP | American Society of Health-System Pharmacists |
| CV | Curriculum vitae |
| IPPE | Introductory pharmacy practice experience |
| MCM | ASHP Midyear Clinical Meeting |
| NMS | National Matching Service |
| PGY1 | Postgraduate year one |
| PGY2 | Postgraduate year two |
| PPS | Personnel Placement Service |
| RPD | Residency program director |
| VA | Department of Veterans Affairs |

## INTRODUCTION

It is an exciting time as you enter your final professional year. At this time, most of the major activities and decisions related to the residency application process will take place. During the year, you will finalize the residency programs you are interested in applying to, complete the application and interview process, and begin the course for your career. The events and accomplishments of the year are the culmination of your hard work and efforts in the previous years. Table 1 provides a timeline of events for researching and applying to residency programs.

**Table 1.** Securing Your Residency: A Timeline for Your Final Professional Year

| | |
|---|---|
| **Pre-fourth year/ summer** | • Optimize clinically based APPEs.<br>• Schedule "off" rotations during February for residency interviews if possible.<br>• Begin APPEs – treat each one as a job interview; volunteer for projects<br>• Identify a project for poster presentation at a professional organization meeting.<br>• Register for ASHP MCM.<br>• Secure hotel reservations for MCM – opens mid-July.<br>• Participate in clinically based competitions hosted by professional organizations. |
| **September** | • Evaluate your APPE progress and update your interests.<br>• Keep a journal/portfolio of interesting patient cases, especially ones in which you played an active role.<br>• Participate in the ACCP Clinical Pharmacy Challenge.<br>• Update CV and ask others to review it.<br>• Submit CV to the ACCP Online CV Review Program for external review and feedback.<br>• Start contemplating contacts to provide letters of reference.<br>• Research and attend available regional residency showcases. |
| **October** | • Attend ACCP Annual Meeting.<br>• Participate in ACCP Residency and Fellowship Forum.<br>• Register for ASHP PPS, if interested.<br>• Early registration deadline for ASHP MCM<br>• Register for ASHP Resident Matching Program "The Match" (https://portal.phorcas.org).<br>• Start developing your letter of interest for the application process. |
| **November** | • Ask colleagues, mentors, and preceptors to read your letter of intent.<br>• Review ASHP MCM Residency Showcase schedule; make a list of programs, and plan a strategy for meeting with programs.<br>• Discuss your list with mentors.<br>• Develop a list of questions you want to ask programs at the showcase.<br>• E-mail residency program directors and tell them you are looking forward to meeting them at the showcase.<br>• Contact programs you would like to meet at PPS to set up an interview time, if applicable.<br>• Finalize contacts to provide letters of reference. |

| | |
|---|---|
| **December** | • Attend MCM.<br>• Write thank you notes to programs of interest spoken to at the residency showcase.<br>• Complete applications for programs.<br>• Request transcripts. |
| **January** | • Submit residency program application by the individual deadlines.<br>• Begin scheduling on-site interviews.<br>• Arrange travel and accommodations.<br>• Contact each preceptor for your January, February, and March APPEs to let them know of your interview plans. |
| **February** | • On-site residency interviews<br>• Send thank you notes after each interview.<br>• Prepare rank list for the match. |
| **March** | • Submit rank order list early in March. Do not wait until the match deadline for submissions (www.natmatch.com/ashprmp/).<br>• Receive match results in mid- to late March. |

ACCP = American College of Clinical Pharmacy; APPE = Advanced Pharmacy Practice Experience; ASHP = American Society of Health-System Pharmacists; CV = curriculum vitae; MCM = (ASHP) Midyear Clinical Meeting; PPS = (ASHP) Personnel Placement Service.

To accomplish the goals you have set for yourself, it is important to stay focused and continue to build experiences. Take full advantage of your Advanced Pharmacy Practice Experiences (APPEs). Treat each one as a job interview throughout the APPE. Go the extra mile when building your therapeutic knowledge base during patient evaluations and clinical presentations as well as when completing your rotational assignments. Make the most of any second-choice APPEs by offering to take on extra projects, writing a newsletter, participating in a committee charge, or giving a drug-related presentation or inservice. When your APPE preceptor is also a residency preceptor or residency program director (RPD), engage him or her in conversations about residency training. Find out what he or she is looking for in a prospective residency candidate and what qualities make a successful resident. Finalize opportunities for research and poster presentation or publication that can be completed this year. Finally, stay involved in professional organizations, and look for additional leadership opportunities that can be completed while on APPEs. Use the resources available for students within professional organizations, such as the American College of Clinical Pharmacy (ACCP) Curriculum Vitae Online Review service, and further develop your clinical skills by entering a student competition. Remember to update your curriculum vitae (CV) with all of your activities and accomplishments throughout the year.

## RESEARCHING RESIDENCY PROGRAMS

If you haven't started already, begin researching potential residency programs at the beginning of your final year in the curriculum. There are more than 975 postgraduate year one (PGY1) residencies to choose from, and narrowing them down to a manageable number for researching may seem like an overwhelming task (References 1–3). To focus your search, it is important to define what you want in a residency, as described in Step I. Keep your goals in mind as you delineate your professional and practice interests.

The first step is to determine what type of residency program to research. The term *PGY1 residency* refers to the first year of training upon graduation, and it is the residency graduating students pursue. In general, these residencies provide more broad-based learning experiences, whereas postgraduate year two (PGY2) residencies are designed for specialized training in a particular area (e.g., ambulatory care, cardiology, infectious diseases). PGY1 residencies accredited by the American Society of Health-System Pharmacists (ASHP) are categorized as pharmacy, community pharmacy, or managed care (Reference 4). The most prevalent programs are PGY1 Pharmacy residencies. They are typically conducted in a hospital, although some programs are primarily administered in an ambulatory clinic or home infusion company. Combined PGY1- and PGY2-accredited programs are also available in areas such as administration and pharmacotherapy.

Graduating students may also choose to pursue nonaccredited residencies. These are commonly offered in a specialized area. Although residents may develop practice or other skills in both accredited and nonaccredited residency programs, accredited programs undergo a peer-review process against a set of optimal standards to ensure the best possible learning experiences. In addition, graduates of accredited residencies are increasingly receiving more recognition among the profession. Examples of this recognition include being eligible for board certification and serving as a residency preceptor or program director sooner than graduates of nonaccredited programs (References 4, 5).

Once you have chosen the type of PGY1 residency to pursue, start reviewing and comparing the characteristics, opportunities, and training philosophy between programs. Consider starting your search through recommendations from mentors, nationally recognized programs, and geographic location; then, branch out from there. If your chosen path is to pursue a community pharmacy, managed care, or a combined PYG1/PGY2 residency program, the number of programs offered is much smaller, and it may be easier to focus your research.

## Program Characteristics
### Institution
To focus your search for PGY1 Pharmacy residency programs offered in hospitals, think about the type of environment that will foster your learning style. Although exceptions occur within distinct hospitals, common themes often emerge related to the training experience. Academic medical centers by definition are affiliated with a college of medicine and usually other health professional schools and colleges, such as pharmacy or nursing (Reference 6). Most are also known for engaging in cutting-edge research. Students and trainees from a variety of disciplines are often present in the patient care units and ambulatory clinics. Patient care rounds are usually interdisciplinary, meaning that physicians, pharmacists, and other health care professionals participate and that a large number of people are involved. The commitment to patient care, number of trainees, and opportunities for research contribute to the teaching and collaborative atmosphere found in most academic medical centers. Academic medical centers are medium to large (300 beds or more) and generally offer specialized care not found in other hospitals. Multidisciplinary teams conduct much of the care provided to patients. The hospital size and specialized services usually provide a variety of learning experiences for pharmacy residents (Reference 7).

Residencies in community hospitals are more prevalent than academic medical centers, and opportunities for resident learning can be quite diverse between institutions. Some community hospitals are designated teaching hospitals that train medical residents as well as other trainees. Some hospitals are quite large and offer a diversity of patient care services. Clinical pharmacists in this setting often work one on one with the physician in the care of patients. The number of preceptors in these programs is usually much smaller, allowing more one-on-one interactions with the preceptors and program directors (Reference 8).

Department of Veterans Affairs (VA) hospitals are unique for the patient population served and pharmacist involvement in the medication use process. The number of inpatient beds varies between institutions, from 50 beds or less to more than 500 beds. Acute care pharmacy services also vary between institutions and depend largely on the number of inpatient beds. Primary care is a strength within the VA system. Pharmacists are recognized as providers within the VA system and are allowed prescriptive authority for medications within their scope of practice (Reference 9). Although the number of women treated within the VA system is growing, most patients are male.

*Academic Affiliation*
Many residency programs have an academic affiliation, or they may be sponsored by a college of pharmacy. The degree of association and teaching opportunities differ between programs. Residents at institutions with an academic affiliation can expect to interact with students on APPEs at a minimum, and some programs offer additional teaching opportunities. Discover what types of teaching the preceptors participate in (experiential teaching of Introductory Pharmacy Practice Experiences [IPPEs] or APPEs, course coordination, laboratory facilitation, recitation, or didactic lecture) and what opportunities are available to the residents. Determine whether any of the preceptors hold full-time, part-time, or adjunct appointments in a college of pharmacy. It is common for programs to offer a teaching certificate program, which provides formal instruction in teaching methods (References 10–12). No standardization for content, requirements, or teaching experiences currently exists among the teaching certificate programs, so you will need to research each individual program, if interested.

*Number of Residents*
Residency class size is another key factor to consider. The smallest PGY1 programs have only one or two residents, whereas the largest programs may have 10 or more residents every year. Candidates looking for one-on-one interaction with the RPD and preceptors that is more direct may opt for a smaller program. Candidates looking for camaraderie and support among their colleagues may be better suited for a larger program. Some programs also include several PGY2 residents, making the total number of residents at the institution quite large (e.g., more than 20). Residents in a small program may report a general ease of scheduling their rotations compared with residents in a large program. Certain pharmacy services and programs may only be found in larger programs with a critical number of residents to deliver the particular service, such as an on-call program or other resident-run services. Institution size does not necessarily predict the number of residents a program will

take. Academic medical centers tend to have larger residency programs and are more likely to offer PGY2 residencies. New residency programs often start with a small number of residents.

*Rotations and Program Requirements*
Candidates may also wish to focus their search on residency programs that offer specific rotations or services based on their interests, such as oncology, pediatrics, or an on-call program. Academic medical centers tend to offer the greatest diversity of rotations, patient population, and specialized services. Community hospitals tend to offer more general medicine–type experiences and specialize in fewer areas (e.g., orthopedic surgery, cardiology, women's health).

In addition to rotation opportunities, programs differ in their fundamental components and minimum requirements to graduate. Although the minimum requirements may be similar among programs, the emphasis placed on individual achievements will vary. For example, a program emphasizing presentation skills may require the completion of a presentation at a professional society meeting or require two grand rounds presentations instead of one. Other programs may require specific teaching activities or emphasize research skills.

*Training Philosophy*
A program's training philosophy encompasses their views and attitudes toward residency training and is one of the most important factors in determining a good fit between candidate and program. Some factors to research and consider include mentorship, evaluation and feedback, practice opportunities, and career paths of past residents. If the program has a formal mentor or adviser program, determine how mentors are assigned to a resident, and learn more about the nature of the relationship with that resident. Ask the current residents about the type and frequency of interaction and feedback they receive from preceptors and mentors.

## Locating Residency Program Information
To begin researching residency programs, use one of the residency directories compiled by professional organizations to identify programs of interest. The ACCP *Directory of Residencies, Fellowships, and Graduate Programs* is published annually and is available both online and in a print version (Reference 2). Each listing provides program contact information, length and type of program, accreditation status, number of residents, salary, and a brief program description. In addition to

accredited and nonaccredited programs, this directory lists fellowships. It is searchable by program type, geographic location, and key word. The accreditation status of each program is included in the listing but is not verified by ACCP. Because the online listings may be updated at any time by the program director or designee, information such as salary, number of residents, and contacts is more likely to be current.

The ASHP Online Residency Directory lists only programs that are accredited or that have applied for accreditation (Reference 3). Each listing provides the program type and length, name of the residency director and program contact, director of pharmacy, number of residents, salary, accreditation status (accredited, candidate, or pre-candidate), a brief description of the program, and institution type, size, and description. Programs may be searched by program type and geographic location. The directory includes an interactive map for locating programs within a specific city, state, or other geographic area.

Once you have identified several programs of interest, the best place to find more detailed information is the program Web site. The Web addresses are listed in the residency directory, and many may also be found through Internet search engines. Often, all recruiting materials, including brochures, are available online. Although the information posted on the program Web sites will vary, information about preceptors, photos of current and past residents, recent awards the program has received, required and elective rotations, and program requirements including staffing and teaching opportunities are often available online.

Candidates may also want to learn more about the preceptors in the program. Preceptors who are also college of pharmacy faculty will often have a faculty Web page describing their professional interests, recent awards, and publications. A more comprehensive and updated list of publications can be found by searching Medline or PubMed. Sometimes, the professional involvement of the preceptors or program director may not be apparent on the program Web site. Performing an Internet search through a search engine may be helpful to identify national or regional involvement on the part of the program preceptors.

After thoroughly reviewing the program materials in the directories, program Web site, and Internet search, speaking with people currently associated with the program or past graduates will provide you with additional information to determine whether the program is a good fit. The main opportunity to talk to the program is at the ASHP Residency Showcase, discussed in the next section. However, other professional organizations and colleges of pharmacy may hold their own national or regional showcases. ACCP holds a Residency and Fellowship Forum at its Annual Meeting held in October. These showcases and forums are an excellent opportunity to talk to prospective programs in a less stressful and less crowded environment.

Seek out individuals who have completed residencies at your college of pharmacy, those whom you encounter on your APPEs, and those at your place of work. Find out where they completed their residency, what they liked about their program, and how they learned about it. Seek mentorship from people whom you aspire to be and from those who share common interests. These mentors are a great source of advice and can play a key role in your professional success.

Candidates may wish to contact the program with additional questions. **Be sure to thoroughly research the program first to avoid asking questions that can be easily found on the Web site or residency directory.** When communicating with the program, remember to keep it professional. Try contacting the program initially by e-mail. All questions posed to the program electronically should be specific. Avoid general questions such as "What can you tell me about your program?" or a long list of questions in an e-mail. If you have a special situation or several questions to ask, do not hesitate to contact the program and request to set up a time to discuss by telephone. If you haven't received a response from the program after a reasonable time has passed (e.g., 1 week), it is okay to contact them again, and the program will probably be grateful, especially if something happened to the first message. Remember, thoughtful, well-researched questions go a long way to making a lasting positive impression on the program.

## PREPARATION FOR THE ASHP MIDYEAR CLINICAL MEETING

The ASHP Midyear Clinical Meeting (MCM) held in December each year is the largest gathering of residency programs and candidates and is a must for those truly interested in pursuing residency training. Meeting attendance has many benefits, chief among which is the opportunity for you as a residency candidate to meet face to face with residency directors, preceptors, and current residents located all across the country. Candidates can speak with prospective programs to determine whether they are interested in devoting time and resources traveling to the specific site. Candidates usually have the opportunity to meet several preceptors and residents who have dedicated time for the purposes of recruiting. Other benefits include the networking and educational opportunities available at the meeting.

Although networking occurs continuously throughout the meeting, ASHP offers two formal opportunities for residency candidates to meet with specific programs, the Residency Showcase and the Personnel Placement Service (PPS). The Residency Showcase is a large exhibit of ASHP-accredited programs (or those seeking accreditation) and serves as a forum for residency candidates and program representatives to meet and discuss individual program opportunities. Because of the number of residencies participating, the showcase is divided into three sessions. The sessions are currently 3 hours long and are typically held on Monday afternoon, Tuesday morning, and Tuesday afternoon of the MCM. Each program is assigned a booth and a number. A directory of programs and a map of the showcase are available on the Web site (www.ashp.org) before the meeting (usually posted in November each year).

If you attended the MCM previously, you have an appreciation for the size of the meeting and number of people in attendance. It can be stressful and somewhat overwhelming experience if you don't know what to expect. It is important to be organized ahead of time. Complete your research on the various residency programs early, and have a list of programs you wish to meet. Make a note of each program's booth number and their scheduled showcase date and time. Consider sending the program director a short e-mail with an attached CV expressing interest in the program; tell the director you are looking forward to learning more about the residency during the showcase. Most programs will appreciate the gesture and will be more likely to remember your name during and after the showcase.

> *As a pharmacy student, I wish I had been given preparatory information regarding the residency showcase and personal placement services. It would have been helpful to understand the interviewing process in regards to PPS and how to navigate the Web site to set up interviews. I would have liked to discuss good questions to ask of current residents and residency directors and fit those responses to the program that would best fit me. It would have been helpful to have assistance in creating a timeline to keep track of everything from when applications were due to when match rankings needed to be submitted.*
>
> —Tammy Berg, 2011/12 PGY2 Pharmacotherapy Resident at Mayo School of Health Sciences, Rochester, Minn.

It can be easy to get overwhelmed when you see the number of interested people outside the exhibit doors, waiting for the showcase to open. Remember to keep your focus on the predetermined plan of programs to meet. The first 20 minutes of the showcase is often the least busy time for residency programs because candidates are trying to find their way around the booths. Most programs will have several residents and preceptors available to talk to candidates. The actual number of people will depend on the size of the program. Some of the most popular programs will have lines of candidates waiting to speak to the preceptors and residents. Candidates can expect to sign in at the booth, leave a copy of their CV, and pick up a copy of the program's recruiting materials (e.g., brochure, CD) if available. Dress in business attire as if you were presenting for an interview.

Although less often used as a recruiting tool for PGY1 residents, some programs also participate in PPS. It, too, is located in a large exhibit hall, but access is restricted to applicants registered separately for this service. Institutions participating in PPS have one or more private booths available for meeting with or interviewing candidates. The main advantage to participating in PPS is the opportunity to schedule a specific time to meet with a program one to one. The list of participating institutions is available to candidates online several weeks before the meeting and is continually updated. The early deadline for PPS is usually October 15 each year. Candidates submit information for an online profile as well as upload a copy of their CV. Candidates have access to registered programs but not to registered applicants. Likewise, programs have access to registered applicants but not to other registered programs. The listing is searchable by several categories, including program type and location. Candidates may contact programs of interest and request an interview. After reviewing the candidate's profile and determining that the candidate is appropriate, programs generally respond to set up a 30-minute interview during the meeting. Although this program is popular among PGY2 programs for recruiting, most PGY1 resident recruiting happens at the Residency Showcase. Before registering for PPS, determine whether any programs you are interested in are participating in PPS by reviewing their Web site or contacting them directly.

In addition to the showcase and PPS, the meeting offers several other residency-related networking opportunities. Attend your state or college of pharmacy reception. Talk to recent graduates from your college of pharmacy who are currently completing a residency. Learn what they like about their program and the type of activities they engage in throughout the year. You may also be invited to attend other receptions by a particular residency program. This is a great opportunity to show your interest in the program.

Beyond residency-related activities, the MCM offers a variety of other events including professional development, educational offerings, business/committee meetings, and industry exhibits. Many networking activities take place during social events. You may catch up with old friends and colleagues, as well as make new friends and acquaintances. It is important to maintain a professional image at all times. If you choose to take any of the complimentary promotional items offered at the industry exhibits, be selective. Limit your alcohol intake during social events. Finally, avoid saying anything negative about a program, classmate, or professor during the meeting because it will reflect poorly on you.

## THE RESIDENCY APPLICATION PROCESS

### The Candidate's Perspective: Choosing Programs for Application

From the candidate's perspective, you should be searching for programs that are a best "fit" for you. Completing these programs will help you achieve your career goals and develop your professional interests in an environment that will foster your growth and learning. Thoughtful research and initial interactions with programs at a regional or national residency showcase will help you identify programs of interest. It is important to conduct a realistic self-appraisal of your skills, abilities, and achievements and to consider the competitiveness of the programs in which you are interested. When deciding on specific programs for application, don't forget practical considerations such as time off APPEs needed to complete on-site interviews and travel costs. The number of interviews you will be able to reasonably complete and the competitiveness of your chosen programs will help you determine how many programs to which you should apply. Table 2 lists several residency application tips and pearls. Beginning in 2013, most ASHP-accredited programs will participate in the Pharmacy Online Residency Centralized Application Service (PhORCAS). The initial fee will allow applicants to upload application materials and submit up to four residency program applications. An additional fee is required for each program application submitted beyond this number. More information is available at https://portal.phorcas.org.

### The Program's Perspective: Selecting Candidates to Interview

From the program's perspective, the RPD and preceptors are also looking for candidates that are the best "fit" for the program. Specifically, programs want residents whose goals and interests match opportunities offered in the residency and who possess characteristics that will help them succeed in the program. Desirable candidate characteristics include therapeutic knowledge, clinical experience, high academic achievements, hospital and other pharmacy-related work experience,

**Table 2.** Residency Application Tips and Pearls

| Do . . . | Don't . . . |
|---|---|
| Treat every APPE as a job interview. | Apply to only a few programs. |
| Show enthusiasm at every interaction with potential residency programs. | Say something negative during the interview. |
| Research potential programs thoroughly. | Be verbose in your letter of intent. |
| Conduct a realistic self-evaluation of your skills and abilities. | Forget to change the last program's contact information when submitting your letter of intent. |
| Ask at least one question of each interviewer or group of interviewers during the on-site interview. | Contact the program and ask a question that is described in its recruiting materials or Web site. |
| Highlight why you would be a good fit for the position. | Forget that you are being evaluated at all times and during all program interactions throughout the application process. |
| Keep a journal of interesting patient cases in which you were actively involved to use as examples during your interviews. | Use emoticons (e.g., smiley face) when communicating with a program. |
| Respond promptly to e-mail messages and provide a professional e-mail address. | Leave your cell phone on during the interview. |
| Eliminate any photos or information that would be considered unprofessional from social networking Web sites. | Carry around bags of "freebies" obtained from the industry exhibits during the Midyear Clinical Meeting. |

APPE = Advanced Pharmacy Practice Experience.

leadership skills, enthusiasm, verbal and written communication skills, and professionalism. The emphasis placed on each of these characteristics by a particular program varies.

In recent years, the number of applications received by individual residency programs has increased dramatically. Because of the financial and personnel resources needed to interview prospective candidates, programs are only able to interview a portion of the qualified candidates. The increase in applications and the need to limit the number of applicants invited for an on-site interview make a candidate's past professional achievements increasingly important. On receipt of residency application materials, the RPD and sometimes one or more preceptors review the application and score the candidate against a predetermined set of criteria. Candidates with the highest rankings are offered an interview. In this process, candidates with the greatest depth and breadth of achievements listed on their CV generally score better. Remember, your CV will serve as your primary representation during the initial candidate evaluation in the residency application process to determine who will be invited for on-site interviews. Because programs rank most of the candidates they interview, getting an interview is the candidate's best chance for obtaining a residency position.

## CHOOSING REFERENCES

Most residency programs require three letters of recommendations written on the candidate's behalf to complete the application. It is your responsibility to identify appropriate people to serve as references and provide the desired information. It is the references' responsibility to provide sufficient detail regarding how well and how long they have known the candidate, in what capacity the references worked with the candidate, the level of support of the candidate for the position, the quality of the candidate's work explained with examples, and the disclosure of any potential conflicts. Some programs may ask references to identify and comment on at least one of the candidate's weaknesses.

Ideal references are those who can provide an honest and detailed account of your professional attributes. As a residency applicant, you want someone to provide a letter in support of your candidacy. It can be challenging to decide which references will provide the best recommendation. Program applications occasionally provide instructions regarding the people from whom they wish to receive recommendations (e.g., a professor, a clinical pharmacist preceptor, and a current or former employer). In this case, it is important to follow these directions and secure these specific individuals to serve as references. If no instructions are given, it is generally best to identify clinical faculty members, preceptors, or other clinical pharmacists with whom you have worked who can comment on your clinical skills. It is not uncommon for residency programs to receive letters of recommendations from college of pharmacy deans or associate deans, directors of pharmacy, managers, or other administrators that provide little detail regarding the candidate's clinical skills or achievements related to the program. Of note, although these people may be well connected within the profession, their support often does little to enhance the candidate's standing without firsthand knowledge and relevant examples of the candidate's professional attributes. Programs also commonly receive recommendations from supervisors or employees that offer not much more information than a few check marks and a statement that the candidate was dependable. Although this type of information does not necessarily reflect negatively on the candidate, it does little to bolster his or her candidacy. Be sure to ask people with significant experience to serve as a reference for you.

When asking someone to serve as a reference or write a letter of recommendation, take the following steps to ensure the best possible outcome. Start by informing your chosen reference author about the programs to which you will be applying. Provide details regarding what you like about the programs and how you believe these programs will help you achieve your career goals. Next, ask whether the individual is able to write a positive letter of recommendation by the stated deadline. This offers a graceful way out if the reference must decline for any reason, such as a conflict of interest or competing deadlines. Provide the individuals agreeing to serve as a reference the following information: (1) program name; (2) institution; (3) name, title, address, and contact information of the RPD or program coordinator to whom the letter should be addressed; (4) an updated copy of your CV; and (5) any information that will assist in writing the letter, such as specific qualities the program is looking for in a candidate (e.g., leadership skills).

## DEVELOPING A LETTER OF INTENT

The purpose of a letter of intent, sometimes also referred to as a cover letter or letter of interest, is to highlight aspects of your CV relative to the position and obtain an invitation to interview. From the program's perspective, the letter of intent is read to determine whether the candidate has the relevant skills, abilities, and experience for the position and good written communication skills and whether the applicant's goals and interests match what the program can offer. This is often the most difficult part of the residency application process for many candidates because they must promote themselves and their achievements. This can feel uncomfortable, especially when just starting out in your career. The key is to substantiate attributes with detailed experiences and to reference specific achievements. For example, describe what you were able to accomplish in your duties as class president rather than simply state that you held this position.

The residency application letter of intent should follow standard business letter format and use a three-paragraph design. Always address the letter to a specific person, usually the RPD or residency coordinator, as indicated in the recruiting materials. It is also very important to read and follow the application instructions, if provided. For example, some programs ask applicants to address specific questions in the letter of intent.

The introductory paragraph should state the position to which you are applying, explain how you heard about the position, and indicate why you are interested. Many letters will reference the MCM or other residency showcase to describe how the candidate learned about the program. In doing so, the program is assured that the candidate has made an effort to seek it out and learn important information that promoted program interest.

The next section, the body of the letter, highlights candidate strengths, achievements, and experiences relevant to the position. Specific examples should be used to illustrate these attributes, and candidates should emphasize relevant achievements from the CV. Be sure to match these skills, strengths, and achievements to each residency for which you are applying. Do not assume that programs will easily recognize achievements listed on your CV. This section is also where the candidate addresses specific questions as indicated in the application instructions. The body is usually one paragraph, but it may include two paragraphs, if needed, to adequately describe candidate qualities or address particular points.

The final paragraph should reinforce interest in the position, indicate why you may be a good fit, and thank the readers for their consideration. This is usually the shortest paragraph in the letter. It is also helpful to indicate an interest in meeting with the program to learn more. It is important to remember that a well-written letter of intent helps candidates receive an invitation for interview but does not secure the position. A sample letter of intent can be found in Appendix 1.

> *I wish I had started on my letter of intent earlier. Composing a solid letter of intent took a decent amount of time, and adding in time for others to review it added even more.*
>
> —Tiffany Pon, 2011/12 PGY1 Pharmacy Practice Resident at University of California, Davis Medical Center, Sacramento, Calif.

When developing your letter of intent, there are several important points to consider. Keep it concise, and avoid being verbose. Do not use bulleted lists in the letter. Most letters of intent should be kept to one page. If you choose to change the font, margins, or font size, be sure the letter can be easily read. A general rule of thumb is to use a font no smaller than 10 point. Keep the font choice professional, such as Times New Roman or Arial. Know the application instructions, and don't assume the same basic letter of intent will suffice for all programs. Finally, ask mentors, classmates, and preceptors to review your letter of intent for clarity and provide comments. Ask them to check the spelling and grammar also, because it is easy to overlook simple errors. Remember that programs view your letter of intent as a demonstration of your writing abilities and communication skills.

## THE INTERVIEW

Congratulations, you have made it to the interview. As you prepare for the interview, keep in mind the purpose of the interview from the candidate's and the program's perspective. During the interview, the candidate is acquiring critical information to determine whether the program is a good fit. It is the candidate's responsibility to communicate his or her interest, motivation, and enthusiasm for the program; relevant clinical and professional experiences; and ability to work with the team. From the program's point-of-view, they are determining whether each candidate is a good fit for the residency and trying to sell the program to prospective candidates. Their job is to answer the following questions for each candidate. (1) Do the program strengths match the candidate's goals and interests? (2) Is the candidate excited about the program and ready to work hard? (3) Will the candidate work well with this team? (4) Does the candidate have the knowledge and skills needed to excel in the program?

The interview itinerary will vary between programs, but some basic characteristics are common to most. Most interviews last ½–1 full day and include a tour of the facility. Most PGY1 programs interview more than one candidate per day. Candidates are often grouped together for a general information session, tour, and lunch. Do not be surprised if you see one of your classmates during an interview or meet new friends or acquaintances that you see again at a different residency interview.

Candidates should wear a conservative professional suit to the interview. A suit coat and pants, a tie, and dress shoes in black, navy, or other dark color are expected for men. Avoid loud or showy patterned suits. Women may wear a dark-colored skirt suit or pantsuit. In general, either is considered acceptable, but the weather may dictate the choice. Pantsuits are often more practical when interviewing in cold climates, especially where there is a lot of snow. Women should also be careful to avoid low-cut or revealing blouses and short skirts. If in doubt, leave it at home. In addition, be prepared to walk long distances, including stairs, and choose shoes accordingly.

Candidates will interview with the RPD, preceptors, current residents, and administrators; other health care professionals may be included as well. The number of preceptors the candidate interviews with will depend on the size of the program. Most residency candidates can expect to participate in three or more separate interview sessions at each PGY1 residency interview (Reference 13). The interview sessions may be scheduled as one to one (candidate to interviewer), a panel (one candidate with several interviewers), or a group (one interviewer with several candidates). The one-to-one and panel interviews are the two most common types of interviews. The panel interview usually causes the most anxiety among candidates. Tips for this type of session include remaining poised, especially in the face of an aggressive interviewer; addressing everyone in the room when asked a question; and asking questions of more than one person as time allows. During the group interview, remember to show courtesy and respect to other candidates at all times, but also make sure you have the chance to answer at least one question.

During the interview sessions, candidates are often asked a combination of reflective questions (e.g., "Why do you want to do a residency?") and experiential questions (e.g., "What was your favorite rotation?"). Although not used by all programs, a common interview technique for experiential questions is the behavior-based interview. This type of interviewing focuses on knowledge, skills, and past experiences associated with residency training to predict future success (Reference 14). Most candidates can expect to answer questions related to reasons for pursuing a residency, pharmacy as a career, and the specific program for which the candidate is interviewing; career goals, practice interests, professional strengths and weaknesses; APPEs; drug therapy recommendations; time management skills; and teamwork. In addition, be prepared to answer questions related to activities or achievements listed in your CV. Two excellent references exist for candidates to review potential interview questions. One is a textbook that includes an exhaustive list of questions you may encounter during any pharmacy-related interview (Reference 15), and the other includes questions that residents reported being asked during their residency interviews (Reference 13).

Clinical competencies or an assessment of candidate knowledge and skills is becoming an increasingly popular part of the interview process (References 13, 16). The activity and administration vary among programs but may include evaluating a clinical study (i.e., journal club), evaluating a patient case, composing a SOAP note, answering clinical questions verbally, giving a presentation on a clinical topic or patient case, and providing written answers to clinical questions or a patient case, among others. Some programs provide the journal club article or patient case before the interview, whereas others give the candidates a predetermined amount of time to review the material or answer questions.

Do not be surprised if the first step toward being invited for an on-site interview includes a telephone, webcam, or other distance technology interview. Although telephone interviews have not traditionally been used extensively in residency interviews, they are becoming more common as the number of applications rises. A directive interview technique is typically used in which all candidates are asked the same questions by the interviewers (Reference 14). This technique allows efficient comparisons between candidates to determine who should be invited for an on-site interview. The same rules apply for telephone and on-site interviews. When communicating by telephone, it is especially important to take the call in a quiet place (e.g., an office with a closed door), confirm the schedule, avoid making distracting noises or interrupting the speaker, and, above all, be prepared. This includes having your list of questions ready, a copy of your CV in front of you, and a copy of any specific program information to which you may want to refer. A common mistake residency applicants make during telephone interviews is giving the impression they are unprepared for the interview.

## WRITING THANK YOU LETTERS

After the interview, candidates should write an individualized letter of appreciation to each program, usually within 3 days of the interview (Reference 17). At a minimum, you should acknowledge the interview and date it occurred, and thank the program for their time and consideration of your candidacy. Well-written thank you notes also express enthusiasm for the position, highlight why the candidate would be a good fit for the program, and reiterate the candidate's interest in the program, if appropriate. Candidates can convey enthusiasm by providing a thoughtful statement about the strengths of the program and highlighting aspects of the program they find appealing. The thank you letter may also be used to address an unresolved item or reiterate an important point. If you really like the program and consider it a good match for you, do not hesitate to communicate your interest in the thank you letter. A simple statement of your interest in the program and for the potential to work with the team will communicate the message. Remember, from the program's perspective, when comparing two or more candidates with similar attributes, the program will want to work with the person who is enthusiastic about the program. A sample thank you letter can be found in Appendix 2.

Thank you letters may be sent to more than one person at the program, but they need not be sent to each person with whom you were introduced. As a general rule, a thank you can be written to each person in the program that you spent significant time with during the interview. Remember to ask for each interviewer's business card during the interview so that you can send thank you notes to individual preceptors as appropriate. Some programs prefer handwritten cards on professional stationery. Some candidates prefer to send thank you letters electronically. If you choose to do this, be sure to include the thank you letter using standard business letter formatting in an attachment, rather than typing the letter in the body of the e-mail message. To avoid formatting and compatibility issues, use the portable document format (PDF) for attachments.

The thank you letter should be concise, of no more than ½–1 page. It is important to be genuine and sincere in the statements you are writing. Avoid making statements that you do not firmly believe. No matter your level of interest in the program, a good thank you letter will include at least one positive aspect about the program. Remember, a well-written thank you will help you maintain a positive lasting impression with the program.

## THE MATCH

The ASHP pharmacy residency matching process, otherwise known as "The Match," is a process whereby both candidates and fully accredited and candidate-status programs are matched to each other through a computerized process on the basis of a rank-ordered list submitted by each. To be included in the match, candidates register with the National Matching Service (NMS), through the Pharmacy Online Residency Centralized Application Service (PhORCAS) (https://portal.phorcas.org), agree to the terms and conditions, pay a fee, and receive a candidate match number (Reference 1). It is a good idea to register early (registration begins in October each year) so that you can include your match number on your CV and residency application materials and can ensure that programs have your match number during the interview. Although programs can look up your number on the NMS Web site, it is helpful to provide your number to verify accuracy.

Once you have completed all of your residency interviews, it is time to rank the programs in order of preference and submit your rank-ordered list to the NMS (Reference 1). Candidates should understand that the match is run in the candidate's favor. With this in mind, it is important to rank programs according to your preference, not how you think programs will rank you. You should not rank programs about which you have considerable reservations or would not be happy, should you be matched with the program. When signing up for the match, candidates agree to accept the results of it. This means that, except in extreme circumstances, you must enter the program with which you are matched. If you had reservations about the program initially, it could be a long and miserable year for you. Finally, do not wait until the last day to input your choices. Because of the number of applications and programs participating, the Web site may run very slow or temporarily shut down, causing a great deal of stress.

From the program's perspective, several groups of people, preceptors, administrators, and residents usually provide recommendations on the program ranking. Although the ultimate decision lies with the RPD, the ranking is rarely, if ever, based on one person's opinion. Most often, key groups of people meet together in smaller groups to discuss the ranking of the candidates. The small group rankings are sent to the RPD or residency advisory committee to make the final list. With this method, you can easily see why it is important to make a good impression, show enthusiasm, and stay engaged with every person you meet from the program. Engaging the RPD or director of pharmacy is not enough to make it on or at the top of the rank list. Candidates ranked first or near the top are the individuals whom almost everyone agrees are excellent candidates.

## How the Match Works

Both the candidate and programs submit their rank-ordered list online by the deadline. The rankings are entered in a computer program that determines the match results. The match process always starts with the candidate's rankings first. If the candidate's first choice is also a first choice for the program, it is a match. If the candidate's first-choice program did not rank him or her first, the computer will run the match of all the program's top choices and confirm matches of each person higher on the rank list before going to the candidate's second choice. A commonly held misconception about the match is that candidates are matched with the program's top choice. Of importance, remember that candidates are

**Table 3.** Top 10 Ways to Increase Your Chances of "Scrambling"

10. Failure to "do your homework"
9. Apply to only a few programs (and only the most competitive ones)
8. Try to guess how the programs will rank you and match accordingly
7. Be "high maintenance" or in general show a lack of flexibility during your interactions with programs
6. Get too "cozy" or come off as arrogant during the interview; say something negative about a rotation, professor, or colleague
5. Show a lack of enthusiasm during the interview or showcase
4. Ask no questions during all or part of the interview
3. Tell the program you are interested in their location
2. Ask what this program can do for you at all of your interviews
1. Commit program "suicide" by ranking only 1 or 2 programs.

matched with the highest program on their rank list that also ranked the candidate. A more detailed explanation of the matching process can be found on the NMS Web site (www.natmatch.com/ashprmp).

## The Scramble

Candidates who don't match with a program may participate in the post-match process or scramble. Beginning in 2013, a list of programs with open positions that were not filled during the match will be made available on the Monday following publication of the match results. Candidates must contact programs of interest and submit all application materials just as they did when applying to programs before the match. Programs and applicants using the PhORCAS prior to the match will use the system during the post-match process. Applicants will be able to upload new materials as needed. Because of the number of available candidates compared with the number of unmatched positions, programs often receive many inquiries and applications. Telephone interviews occur often in the post-match scramble, and most programs require an on-site interview as well. If you find yourself in this situation, it is a good idea to reach out to your college of pharmacy professors, preceptors, and mentors for help in sorting through the list and receiving guidance on the programs with positions available.

## Increase Your Chances of Matching with a Residency Program

The best thing you can do to secure a residency position beyond following the advice detailed in this book is to complete several on-site interviews. Programs rank most of the candidates they bring in for an interview. Rarely do programs match with all the candidates at the top of their list, and candidates do not know where they rank on the list because of the confidential nature of the ranking process. During the interview, ask thoughtful questions, engage your interviewers, make connections with the program preceptors, and show enthusiasm at all times for the program. Show them you have done your research on the program. After the interview, follow up with well-written thank you notes. State the reasons you are excited about the program, and let them know of your interest in the program. Remember, when programs have several equally qualified candidates, they will choose those who are excited to join their program, are willing to work hard, and enjoy what they do. Table 3 lists several behaviors that commonly cause residency candidates not to be ranked by a program.

## CONCLUSION

The final professional year is both an exciting and important time. One of the most significant events is preparing for and successfully matching with a residency program that will strengthen and advance you as a clinician and foster your continued excellence as a health care provider. Your residency program will also provide a foundation that you will continue to build on throughout your career. To this end, this chapter provides and outlines each of the key responsibilities and activities you must accomplish in your last year as a pharmacy student to become a resident. It is time to step up to the plate and maximize what you have and will accomplish in your last year that will make you competitive for the residency program you desire. Keep a clear focus and enthusiasm as you work toward your goal. Continue to build experiences, finalize your CV, decide which programs you will apply to, choose references, apply to programs, complete interviews, and participate in the match. The hard work you have completed, researching programs and developing a compelling letter of intent, will pay off during the interview and match process. Your steadfast follow-through on each key step will help you obtain a residency position that best fits you.

## ACKNOWLEDGMENT

*The author would like to thank Kelly Martin, Pharm.D., BCPS, for her participation and willingness to share the letter of intent example with the readers of this book.*

## REFERENCES

1. ASHP Resident Matching Program. Summary of Programs and Positions Offered and Filled by Program Type for the 2012 Match. Available at www.natmatch.com/ashprmp/. Accessed August 22, 2012.
2. American College of Clinical Pharmacy. 2012 Directory of Residencies, Fellowships, and Graduate Programs. Lenexa, KS: American College of Clinical Pharmacy, 2011.
3. ASHP Online Residency Directory. Available at http://accred.ashp.org/aps/pages/directory/residencyProgramSearch.aspx. Accessed August 22, 2012.
4. American Society of Health System-Pharmacists. Residency Accreditation Regulations and Standards. Available at www.ashp.org/menu/Accreditation/ResidencyAccreditation.aspx#RegulationsandStandards. Accessed August 22, 2012.
5. Board of Pharmaceutical Specialties. 2012 Candidate's Guide. Available at www.bpsweb.org/pdfs/CandidatesGuide.pdf. Accessed August 22, 2012.
6. Wartman SA. The Academic Health Center: Evolving Organizational Models. The Association of Academic Health Centers. Available at www.aahcdc.org/Portals/0/pdf/AAHC_Evolving_Organizational_Models.pdf. Accessed August 22, 2012.
7. Phillips H, Jasiak KD, Lindberg LS, et al. Characteristics of postgraduate year 1 pharmacy residency programs at academic medical centers. Am J Health Syst Pharm 2011;68:1437-42.
8. Paciullo CA, Moranville MP, Suffoletta TJ. Pharmacy practice residency program in community hospitals. Am J Health Syst Pharm 2009;66:536-9.
9. Cone SM, Brown MC, Stambaugh RL. Characteristics of ambulatory care clinics and pharmacists in Veterans Affairs medical centers: an update. Am J Health Syst Pharm 2008;65:631-5.
10. Romanelli F, Smith KM, Brandt BF. Teaching residents how to teach: a scholarship of teaching and learning certificate program (STLC) for pharmacy residents. Am J Pharm Educ 2005;69:126-32.
11. Castellani V, Haber SL, Ellis SC. Evaluation of a teaching certificate program for pharmacy residents. Am J Health Syst Pharm 2003;60:1037-41.
12. Gettig JP, Sheehan AH. Perceived value of a pharmacy resident teaching certificate program. Am J Pharm Educ 2008;72:article 104.
13. Reinders TP. Introduction to searching and interviewing. In: Reinders TP, ed. The Pharmacy Professional's Guide to Resumes, CVs and Interviewing, 3rd ed. Washington, DC: American Pharmacists Association, 2011:97-104.
14. Mancuso CE, Paloucek FP. Understanding and preparing for pharmacy practice residency interviews. Am J Health Syst Pharm 2004;61:1686-9.
15. Reinders TP. Interview Questions. In: Reinders TP, ed. The Pharmacy Professional's Guide to Resumes, CVs and Interviewing, 3rd ed. Washington, DC: American Pharmacists Association, 2011:111-30.
16. Mersfelder TL, Bickel RJ. Structure of postgraduate year 1 pharmacy residency interviews. Am J Health Syst Pharm 2009;66:1075-6.
17. Reinders TP. Types of letters. In: Reinders TP, ed. The Pharmacy Professional's Guide to Resumes, CVs and Interviewing, 3rd ed. Washington, DC: American Pharmacists Association, 2011:131-3.

# APPENDIX 1

**Tracy White**
735 Baldwin Street
Baltimore, MD 21230
twhite@email.com

December 28, 20XX

John Smith, Pharm.D., BCOP
University Hospital, Department of Pharmacy
200 Hospital Circle
XX, XX

Dear Dr. Smith:

I had the pleasure of speaking with your colleagues and several current PGY1 and PGY2 residents at the Residency Showcase and am writing to express my interest in the University Hospital PGY1 residency program. I am very impressed with the diversity of rotational opportunities offered, the number of board-certified pharmacists serving as preceptors, the on-call program, and the formalized teaching certificate program. I am confident a residency at University Hospital would facilitate my independence as a clinician and guide me to become a leader in the pharmacy profession.

During my second year in pharmacy school, I was honored to be selected for the Veterans Affairs Learning Opportunities Residency, a competitive program in which I was exposed to both hospital and clinical pharmacy, allowing me to experience the progressive practice of pharmacy in the VA system. Inspired by this experience, I selected demanding didactic electives and clerkship experiences in critical care, internal medicine, and cardiology to continue to develop my clinical skills that will prepare me for residency training. On completion of a PGY1, I plan to pursue a specialized residency, become board certified in pharmacotherapy, and practice as a faculty member at a school of pharmacy. I believe the residency program at University Hospital will provide me with the experiences in acute care and ambulatory care that I will need as a foundation to reach my career goals.

Several experiences have strengthened my passion for teaching, including formally tutoring my peers, participating in the Student Committee on Drug Abuse Education, attending the American Association of Colleges of Pharmacy meeting as a Walmart Scholar, and completing a teaching clerkship as a P4. I plan to apply for the teaching certificate program, which will provide me with formalized training and teaching opportunities, allowing me to develop a portfolio and giving me the necessary background to competitively pursue a position in academia. Furthermore, I believe research is an integral part of clinical pharmacy, and I hope to conduct research throughout my career.

My involvement in research began as an undergraduate at Cornell University, and I have continued to develop a wide range of research skills in pharmacy school, recently submitting two applications to the human institutional review board in different states. University Hospital's Residency Research Committee and the requirement to submit a manuscript for publication demonstrate the program's commitment to quality research, and I feel I would greatly benefit from this aspect of the program.

University Hospital's residency program will provide broad, diverse experiences and superb mentoring that will help me achieve my career goals of becoming not only a clinician, educator, and researcher but also a leader in pharmacy, as the program has a reputation of producing excellent pharmacists. Thank you for your time and consideration, and I look forward to hearing from you regarding my application.

Sincerely,


Tracy White

# APPENDIX 2

Amy Reynolds
1528 Baker Street
Portland, OR 97201

February 7, 20XX

Dear Dr. Jones:

Thank you for the opportunity to interview for the PGY1 Residency at Regional Medical Center on February 4. I enjoyed meeting you and the program's preceptors during the interview to learn more about the program. Each individual I met throughout the day spoke enthusiastically of what I continue to believe is an exemplary residency program. It was evident to me that the program provides the resident with a well-rounded training environment through a wealth of clinical experiences, teaching opportunities, and the philosophy of allowing a resident room to further develop into a confident, independent practitioner with the skills necessary to be successful in any post-residency endeavor. I am very excited about the opportunities this program provides, and I have no doubt it would provide a solid training experience that would allow me to fulfill my goal of becoming a competent clinical pharmacist and eventual faculty member at a school of pharmacy. I hope to work with you in the future.

Sincerely,


Amy Reynolds

# CONTRIBUTORS

Jerry L. Bauman, Pharm.D., FCCP, FACC
University of Illinois at Chicago
College of Pharmacy
Chicago, Illinois

Stephen F. Eckel, Pharm.D., MHA, BCPS
University of North Carolina Hospitals
UNC Eshelman School of Pharmacy
Chapel Hill, North Carolina

Janet P. Engle, Pharm.D., FAPhA
University of Illinois at Chicago
College of Pharmacy
Chicago, Illinois

Brian L. Erstad, Pharm.D., FCCP, BCPS
University of Arizona
College of Pharmacy
Tucson, Arizona

Stuart T. Haines, Pharm.D., FCCP, BCPS, BCACP
University of Maryland
School of Pharmacy
Baltimore, Maryland

Dana P. Hammer, R.Ph., M.S., Ph.D.
University of Washington
School of Pharmacy
Seattle, Washington

Marcella Hoyland, Pharm.D., BCPS
University of Arizona
College of Pharmacy
Tucson, Arizona

Donald E. Letendre, Pharm.D.
University of Iowa
College of Pharmacy
Iowa City, Iowa

Erin M. Nystrom, Pharm.D., BCNSP
Mayo Clinic
Rochester, Minnesota

Brandon J. Patterson, Pharm.D.
University of Iowa
College of Pharmacy
Iowa City, Iowa

Heather A. Personett, Pharm.D., BCPS
Mayo Clinic
Rochester, Minnesota

Beth Bryles Phillips, Pharm.D., FCCP, BCPS
University of Georgia
College of Pharmacy
Athens, Georgia

Garrett E. Schramm, Pharm.D., BCPS
Mayo Clinic
Rochester, Minnesota

Keri A. Sims, Pharm.D., BCPS
American College of Clinical Pharmacy
Lenexa, Kansas

# REVIEWERS

The American College of Clinical Pharmacy, the editors, and the authors would like to thank the following individuals for their careful review.

Bradley A. Boucher, Pharm.D., FCCP, BCPS
*University of TennesSee*
*Memphis, TennesSee*

Curtis E. Haas, Pharm.D., FCCP, BCPS
*University of Rochester Medical Center*
*Rochester, New York*

Brian A. Hemstreet, Pharm.D., FCCP, BCPS
*University of Colorado*
*Skaggs School of Pharmacy and*
*   Pharmaceutical Sciences*
*Aurora, Colorado*

Michelle L. Kucera, Pharm.D., BCPS
*American College of Clinical Pharmacy*
*Lenexa, Kansas*

Joseph Lassiter, Pharm.D., M.S., BCPS
*Pacific University*
*School of Pharmacy*
*Hillsboro, Oregon*

Robert B. Parker II, Pharm.D., FCCP
*University of TennesSee*
*College of Pharmacy*
*Memphis, TennesSee*

Cynthia A. Sanoski, Pharm.D., FCCP, BCPS
*Thomas Jefferson University*
*Jefferson School of Pharmacy*
*Philadelphia, Pennsylvania*

Robert E. Smith, Pharm.D.
*Auburn University*
*Harrison School of Pharmacy*
*Auburn University, Alabama*

Rachel C. Stratman, Pharm.D., BCPS
*Barnes-Jewish Hospital*
*St. Louis, Missouri*

James E. Tisdale, Pharm.D., FCCP, FAPhA, FAHA, BCPS
*Purdue University*
*College of Pharmacy*
*Indianapolis, Indiana*

Thomas D. Zlatic, Ph.D.
*St. Louis College of Pharmacy*
*St. Louis, Missouri*

# INDEX

Page numbers followed by b, f, or t indicate material in boxes, figures, or tables, respectively.

## A

abstract, writing and submission of, 140
academic affiliation, of residency programs, 172
academic medical centers, 171, 173
academic record, 15. *See also* grades
academic rotation, 80
Academy of Managed Care Pharmacy (AMCP), 50t
ACCP. *See* American College of Clinical Pharmacy
Accreditation Council for Pharmacy Education (ACPE), 32, 76, 90, 159
accredited residency programs, 170, 178
ACPE. *See* Accreditation Council for Pharmacy Education
action plans, 4–10, 66, 69–70, 71t
action-taking, in time management, 66, 68
action verbs, on curriculum vitae, 156, 157t
activities. *See* involvement
advanced pharmacy practice experiences (APPEs), 27–28, 89–113
   academic (teaching and research), 80
   assessment in, 107–8, 119
   communication in
     with health care team, 102–4
     with patient, 97–100
     with preceptor, 96–97, 98b, 99b, 106–7
   critical thinking and understanding in, 93–95
   failed rotation in, consequences of, 91
   interdisciplinary activities in, 102–5
   interdisciplinary rounding in, 105–6
   introduction to site, 96–97
   as investment in own education, 90–91
   and letters of recommendation, 91, 95, 108–9
   maximizing experience in, 89–90, 109, 110b–111b, 169–70
   networking in, 119–20
   patient care in, 97–107
     discussions with preceptors about, 106–7
     as focus, 94–95, 97–100
     frustration over recommendation not taken, 104–5
     interdisciplinary, 100–106
     pharmacy students as contributors to, 102
   perceptions of pharmacy students in, 105–6
   pre-rotation preparation for, 96
   professionalism in, 91–93
   progression from IPPE to, 94–95
   relationship with preceptor in, 97, 98b
   research ideas from, 131–32
   resources for, 108
   scheduling and selecting rotations in, 95
   settings for, 76–77, 90–91
   student engagement in, 77
   successful, 109, 110b–111b
   work experience in, 76–78
advisor. *See* mentor(s)

Alpha Zeta Omega, 51t
altruism, 130–31
AMCP. *See* Academy of Managed Care Pharmacy
American Association of Colleges of Pharmacy, 108
American College of Cardiology, 140
American College of Clinical Pharmacy (ACCP), vii, viii, 22, 45, 46t, 49t, 50t, 122, 168t
   Curriculum Vitae Online Review, 161, 169–70
   *Directory of Residencies, Fellowships, and Graduate Programs*, 173–74
   Residency and Fellowship Forum, 174–75
*American Journal of Pharmaceutical Education*, 108
American Pharmacists Association (APhA), 49, 50t
American Pharmacists Association Academy of Student Pharmacists (APhA-ASP), 45, 52
American Society of Health-System Pharmacists (ASHP), 50t
   abstract submission to, 140
   involvement in, 41, 50t
   The Match, 150, 186–89
   Midyear Clinical Meeting, 77–78, 175–78
   online group of, 49
   Online Residency Directory, 174
   Personnel Placement Service, 176–77
   PGY1 residencies accredited by, 170
   Residency Showcase, 77–78, 174, 176–77
amiodarone clinic study, 138
APhA. *See* American Pharmacists Association
APhA-ASP. *See* American Pharmacists Association Academy of Student Pharmacists
APPEs. *See* advanced pharmacy practice experiences
application process, 15, 178–92. *See also* candidates
   candidate's perspective on, 178
   choosing references for, 180–81
   interview in, 183–85
   letter of intent for, 181–83, 190–91
   The Match in, 150, 186–89
   program's perspective on, 178–80
   score and ranking in, 179–80
   selection for interview in, 178–80
   timeline for, 120, 168t–169t
   tips and pearls on, 179t
ASHP. *See* American Society of Health-System Pharmacists
assessment
   in experiential education, 107–8, 119
   grades in. *See* grades
   in interview for residency, 184–85
assignable goals, 66–67, 66t
attainable goals, 7–10, 8b–9b
authoritarian leaders, 19t
awards, on curriculum vitae, 157

## B

balance, 38–39
  and experiential education, 90
  and project management, 70
  and time management, 66, 68, 83
  and well-rounded candidacy, 43
  and work experience, 83, 87
behavioral-based interviewing, 84–85, 85b
Big L versus little l's, 58, 60–61

## C

candidates
  academic record (grades) of, 15, 27–28, 32–39
  application process for, 15, 120, 178–92
  community and professional involvement of, 41–54
  desirable, qualities of, 178–79
  experiential education of, 27–28, 76–78, 80, 89–113
  interview of, 183–84, 189
  leadership skills/experience of, 18, 41–42, 57–64, 72–73
  letter of intent, 181–83, 190–91
  letters of recommendation, 91, 95, 108–9, 113–15, 130, 180–81
  management skills of, 57–58, 64–73
  The Match for, 150, 186–89
  Midyear Clinical Meeting for, 77–78, 175–78
  networking by, 43, 81–82, 113–27
  nongraded transcripts of, 35–37
  numbers of, 15, 149–50
  portfolio of, 36–37, 44
  preparation of, 15–20, 22t–23t, 24, 38, 149
  research/scholarship by, 80, 129–45
  selection for interview, 178–80
  thank you letters from, 185–86, 189, 192
  tips and pearls for, 179t
  training options for, 14–15, 16t–17t, 170
  work experience of, 19, 75–87
career-building activities, 15–20, 22t–23t
career plan, 14–20
case reports, 144
certifications, on curriculum vitae, 155
change agents, 57–58, 63–64
clinical practice guidelines, 108
clinical research, 138–39
coaching, as leadership style, 19t
collective leadership, 58, 60–61
communication
  curriculum vitae for, 151–52
  grades as means of, 33
  with health care team, 102–4
    defensive position in, 103–4
    direct versus subtle approach, 103
    methods to avoid, 103
  in networking, 123–25
  with patients, 97–100
  with preceptor, 96–97, 98b, 99b, 106–7
  with residency program, 175
community activities, 52–54
  on curriculum vitae, 157
  involvement in, 41–44
  networking in, 43, 119
community hospital residencies, 171
community pharmacy
  experiential education in, 76, 90–91
  work experience in, 75–76, 78
community pharmacy PGY1 residency, 170
confidence, 38, 81, 108, 150–51
continuing pharmacy education (CPE), 30–32
continuing professional development (CPD), 30–32
  continuous versus episodic, 31
  cycle of, 31, 32f
Costa, Arthur, 13
cover letter, 181–83, 190–91
Covey, Franklin, 6b
Covey, Stephen, 13, 67–68
CPD. *See* continuing professional development
CPE. *See* continuing pharmacy education
credibility, 37–38
critical thinking, 93–95
*Crossing the Quality Chasm: A New Healthcare System for the 21st Century* (Institute of Medicine), 100–101
curbside consult, 122
curriculum vitae (CV), 150–65
  accomplished confidence for, 150–51
  ACCP program on, 161, 169–70
  action verbs on, 156, 157t
  for applicants from nongraded programs, 36–37
  desirable, qualities of, 152–53, 153t
  directed message of, 151
  education on, 155
  electronic submission of, 158
  elements to avoid, 158–59
  emotional introspection on, 150–51
  employment and professional experience on, 155–56
  font for, 158–59
  headings on, 154, 154b
  honors and awards on, 157
  importance of, 150
  layout and content of, 153–56
  length of, 150
  letter of intent with, 181–83, 190–91
  licensures and certifications on, 155
  origin of term, 150
  personal information on, 154–55
  presentations, research, and publications on, 156
  professional activities on, 44, 157
  proofreading of, 158
  references/recommendations on, 109
  versus resume, 150
  review and update of, 169–70
  sample of, 162–65
  targeted audience for, 151–52
  volunteering and community service on, 157

## D

data analysis
  in completion of research, 139
  of existing data, research through, 136–37
defensive position, 103–4
delegation, 71–72
democratic leadership, 19t
design, of research project, 135–39
digoxin studies, 136–37
directive leaders, 63
*Directory of Residencies, Fellowships, and Graduate Programs* (ACCP), 173–74
distance technology interview, 185
documentation, 149–65. *See also* curriculum vitae; portfolio
  of involvement in professional organizations, 44–45
  of networking contacts, 125
dress, for interview, 183
drug information resources, 105, 108
Dweck, Carol, 10–12

## E

effective students, characteristics of, 97, 98b
elective rotations, 95
emotional introspection, 150–51
*Endurance* (Lansing), 59–60
e-professionalism, 126–27
etiquette. *See also* professionalism
  in interdisciplinary rounding, 105
evaluation
  of continuing professional development, 31
  of project, 71–72
  of student work (grades), 32
evidence-based medicine, 105
expedited review, 136
experiential education, 27–28, 89–113
  academic (teaching and research), 80
  ACPE recommendations on, 90
  assessment in, 107–8, 119
  communication in
    with health care team, 102–4
    with patient, 97–100
    with preceptor, 96–97, 98b, 99b, 106–7
  critical thinking and understanding in, 93–95
  failed rotation in, consequences of, 91
  interdisciplinary activities in, 102–5
  interdisciplinary rounding in, 105–6
  introduction to site, 96–97
  as investment in own education, 90–91
  IPPE to APPE progression, 94–95
  and letters of recommendation, 91, 95, 108–9
  maximizing experience in, 89–90, 109, 110b–111b, 169–70
  networking in, 119–20
  patient care in, 97–107
    discussions with preceptors about, 106–7
    as focus, 94–95, 97–100
    frustration over recommendation not taken, 104–5
  interdisciplinary, 100–106
    pharmacy students as contributors to, 102
    perceptions of pharmacy students in, 105–6
    pre-rotation preparation for, 96
    professionalism in, 91–93
    relationship with preceptor in, 97, 98b
    research ideas from, 131–32
    resources for, 108
    scheduling and selecting rotations in, 95
    settings for, 76–77, 90–91
    student engagement in, 77
    successful, 109, 110b–111b
    work experience in, 76–78
experiential questions, in interview, 184

## F

Facebook, 49, 126–27
failure, response to, 11, 12b
fellowships, 16t–17t, 173–75
final professional year. *See also* application process
  Midyear Clinical Meeting during, 175–78
  timeline for, 168t–169t
fixed mindset, 10–11, 12b
font
  for curriculum vitae, 158–59
  for letter of intent, 182
fraternities, 45, 51t

## G

galley proof, 143
goal(s)
  annual review of, 10
  challenge of achieving, 38
  as commitment, not obligation, 9–10
  habits of mind and, 10, 13–14, 13b
  help for achieving, 38–39
  mindset and, 10–14
  in project management, 69–70, 71t
  SMART, 7–10, 8b–9b, 66–67, 66t, 69
  in time management, 66–67, 66t
GPA. *See* grades
grades, 32–39
  high, reasons for obtaining, 37–38
  importance of, 33–37
  personality and, 33
  as predictor of success, 34
  programs that do not award, 35–37
  relationship to learning, 27–28, 32–33, 37–38
  in resident selection process, 34–37, 39
  subjectivity of, 33
  work experience and, 81, 83
graduate degree, 16t–17t
growth mindset, 10–14, 15
  definition of, 11
  versus fixed mindset, 11, 12b

## H

habits of mind, 10, 13–14, 13b
headings, on curriculum vitae, 154, 154b
health fairs, 52
Henderson-Hasselbalch equation, 130

honors, on curriculum vitae, 157
honor societies, 48, 51t
hospitals
  experiential education in, 76, 90–91
  settings for residency programs, 171–72
  work experience in, 77, 78
human resources frame leaders, 62
hypothesis-generating research, 139

## I

impact factor (IF), of journals, 141–43
importance, in time management matrix, 67–68
*Index Medicus*, 156
Institute of Medicine (IOM), 100–101
institutional review board (IRB), 135, 136, 137, 138–39, 144
intent, letter of, 181–83, 190–91
interdisciplinary patient care, 100–106
  Institute of Medicine on, 100–101
  nurturing team relationships in, 101–2
  pharmacy students as contributors to, 102
interdisciplinary rounding, 105–6, 171
interest, letter of, 181–83, 190–91
internship, 76, 78, 79, 83, 155
interpersonal management, 65, 69
interview
  behavioral-based, 84–85, 85b
  experience with, 81b, 84–85
  for residency, 183–85
    assessment of competencies and knowledge in, 184–85
    basic characteristics of, 183
    candidate's responsibility in, 183
    distance technology for, 185
    dressing for, 183
    experiential questions in, 184
    and increasing chances for Match, 189
    program's perspective in, 183
    reflective questions in, 184
    selection for, 178–80
    thank you letters after, 185–86, 189, 192
intravenous fluid stability study, 129–30, 137
introductory pharmacy practice experiences (IPPEs), 27–28, 89–113
  ACPE recommendations on, 90
  assessment in, 107–8, 119
  career overview in, 77
  communication in
    with health care team, 102–4
    with patient, 97–100
    with preceptor, 96–97, 98b, 99b, 106–7
  critical thinking and understanding in, 93–95
  failed rotation in, consequences of, 91
  interdisciplinary activities in, 102–5
  interdisciplinary rounding in, 105–6
  introduction to site, 96–97
  as investment in own education, 90–91
  and letters of recommendation, 91, 95, 108–9
  maximizing experience in, 89–90, 109, 110b–111b
  networking in, 119–20
  patient care in, 97–107
    discussions with preceptors about, 106–7
    as focus, 97–100
    frustration over recommendation not taken, 104–5
    interdisciplinary, 100–106
    pharmacy students as contributors to, 102
    perceptions of pharmacy students in, 105–6
    pre-rotation preparation for, 96
  professionalism in, 91–93
  progression to APPE, 94–95
  relationship with preceptor in, 97, 98b
  research ideas from, 131–32
  resources for, 108
  scheduling and selecting rotations in, 95
  successful, 109, 110b–111b
  work experience in, 76–78
in vitro studies, 137
involvement, 41–54
  benefits of, 41–44
  conduct in, 53–54
  constraints on, 45
  importance of, 41
  learning through, 42–43
  making time for, 41, 49
  online resources/opportunities, 49
  strategy for, 48–52
  year-by-year plan for, 44, 46t–47t
IOM. *See* Institute of Medicine
IPPEs. *See* introductory pharmacy practice experiences
IRB. *See* institutional review board

## J

journals
  galley proof for, 143
  general writing guidelines for, 143f
  impact factor of, 141–43
  Instructions for Authors, 141
  revision for, 143
  writing and submitting paper for, 141–43

## K

Kappa Epsilon, 51t
Kappa Psi, 51t

## L

laissez-faire leaders, 19t
Lambda Kappa Sigma, 51t
leadership, 58–64
  Big L versus little l's in, 58, 60–61
  change agents in, 57–58, 63–64
  developing skills of, 57–64
  gaining experience in, 18, 41–42, 44, 72–73
  human resources, 62
  learning precepts of, 59
  versus management, 64
  organizational frames approach to, 62–63

ownership and, 59
philosophy of, 61–63
political, 62–63
principles of, 60
privilege and responsibility of, 59–60
self-initiative in, 61
structural, 62
student, recommended activities for, 72 73, 72t
styles of, 18, 19t, 63
symbolic, 62–63
learning
   in community/professional involvement, 42–43
   experiential, 76–78, 89–113
   lifelong, 30–32
   maximizing opportunities for, 37–38
   relationship of grades to, 27–28, 32–33, 37–38
   self-directed, 28–30
   service, 53
letter of intent, 181–83, 190–91
letters of recommendation, 180–81
   asking for, 181
   experiential education and, 91, 95, 108–9, 119
   information for writers of, 181
   networking and, 113–15, 119
   research/scholarship and, 130
licensures
   on curriculum vitae, 155
   work experience and, 76, 81b, 83
lifelong learning, 30–32
literature search, on research topic, 133–34
local associations, 45–48

## M

managed care PGY1 residency, 170
management, 57–58, 64–73
   depth of, 70
   functions and levels of, 64–65
   versus leadership, 64
   project, 65, 66t, 69–72
   self-, 10–14, 65–72
   strategies and tactics of, 66t
   student, recommended activities for, 72–73, 72t
   time, 39, 65–68, 66t
management skills, development of, 57–73
The Match, 186–89
   failure to obtain, 150, 188, 188t
   improving chances in, 188–89
   number of candidates seeking, 150
   rankings by candidates and programs in, 187–88
   registration for, 186
MCM. *See* Midyear Clinical Meeting
measurable goals, 7–10, 8b–9b
medication use evaluation, 138
Medline, 174
meetings
   professional
      networking in, 120–22
      platform or poster presentation for, 140–41, 142f
      writing and submitting abstract for, 140
   in project management, 71–72

mentor(s)
   age of, 21
   community/professional involvement and, 43, 48, 49
   finding, 20–24
   gender of, 21–24
   letters of recommendation from, 113
   mindset of, 13
   mutual benefits of, 20
   networking and, 116
   personal mission statement of, 6b
   preassigned, switching from, 21
   for research project, 132–35, 141
meta-analysis, 136–37
Midyear Clinical Meeting (ASHP), 77–78, 175–78
mindful practice, 13–14
mindset, 10–14
   definition of, 10
   fixed, 10–11, 12b
   growth, 10–14, 12b, 15
   survey for determining, 12–13
mission statement, personal, 4–7, 6b
Mission Statement Builder, 6b
mock scenarios, for interdisciplinary activities, 102
motivation, grades and, 33

## N

National Community Pharmacists Association (NCPA), 45, 51t
National Library of Medicine, 156
National Matching Service (NMS), 150, 186–87
NCPA. *See* National Community Pharmacists Association
networking, 113–27
   community/professional involvement and, 43, 119, 120–22
   experiential education and, 119–20
   informal, 125–26
   institution-specific, 115–16
   keeping track of contacts, 125
   at Midyear Clinical Meeting, 175–78
   on-campus, 117–19
   online, 49, 126–27
   opportunities for, 116–23, 117f
   plan or strategy for, 123–25
   process of (how to), 123–26
   in professional meetings, 120–22
   shadowing and, 122–23
   timeline for, 114t–115t
   value of, 113–16
   work experience and, 81–82, 81b
*New England Journal of Medicine*, 129, 141
NMS. *See* National Matching Service
nonaccredited residency programs, 170
nongraded transcripts, 35–37
nontenure-track faculty, 134–35

## O

objectives, in project management, 69–70, 71t
observational studies, 136, 139

OEE. *See* Office of Experiential Education
Office of Experiential Education (OEE), 93, 96
office of student affairs, 39
one-to-one interview, 184
online networks, 49, 126–27
Online Residency Directory (ASHP), 174
open positions, after Match, 188
Operation Immunization, 52
optimal patient care, 37
oral platform presentation, 140–41
organization, grades and, 33
organizational frames approach, 62–63
organizational managers, 65
outreach activities, 52
ownership, by leaders, 59

## P

panel interview, 184
participative leaders, 63
passion, 2–10
   aligned with skills and talents, 3–10, 3f
   definition of, 2
   inventory of, 5b
pass/no pass, 35
patient care
   in experiential education, 97–107
      discussions with preceptor about, 106–7
      as focus, 94–95, 97–100
      frustration over recommendation not taken, 104–5
      interdisciplinary, 100–106
      Institute of Medicine on, 100–101
      nurturing team relationships in, 101–2
      pharmacy students as contributors to, 102
   optimal, 37
patient care projects, 52
personal information, on curriculum vitae, 153–54
personal mission statement, 4–7, 6b
personal satisfaction, 38
Personnel Placement Service (PPS), 176–77
pharmacoeconomic analysis, 136–37
pharmacoepidemiologic studies, 136
Pharmacy and Therapeutics Committee, 139
Pharmacy Online Residency Centralized Application Service (PhORCAS), 178, 186, 188
pharmacy practice research, 130
pharmacy technicians, 75
phenytoin stability study, 129–30, 137
Phi Delta Chi, 51t
Phi Lambda Sigma, 48, 51t
philosophy of leadership, 61–63
philosophy of life, 10. *See also* mindset
philosophy of training, 173
PhORCAS. *See* Pharmacy Online Residency Centralized Application Service
plan of action, 4–10, 66, 69–70, 71t
platform presentation, 140–41
political leaders, 62–63
portfolio
   for applicants from nongraded programs, 36–37

professional activities and, 44
residency application, 159–60
Web-based, 36–37
poster presentations, 121, 140–41, 142f
postgraduate training, options for, 14–15, 16t–17t, 170
postgraduate year one (PGY1), 14–15, 16t–17t. *See also* residency program(s)
   definition of, 170
   leadership experiences in, 41–42
   practice-related project in, 130
   researching programs, 170–75
postgraduate year two (PGY2), 15, 16t–17t, 170. *See also* residency program(s)
PPS. *See* Personnel Placement Service
practice evaluation projects, 138–39
practice guidelines, 108
practice-related project, 130
preceptors
   assessment by, 107–8, 119
   discussing patient care with, 106–7
   effective, characteristics of, 97
   expectations in IPPE versus APPE, 94–95
   information discussed with/provided by, 97, 99b
   introduction/orientation by, 96–97
   learning about, 174
   letters of recommendation from, 91, 95, 108–9, 119
   networking with, 119–20
   opportunities in residency programs, 172
   pre-rotation contact with, 96
   professionalism of, 92–93
   relationship with, tips for effective, 97, 98b
prioritization, 66, 67–68
professionalism
   in experiential education, 91–93
   in online networking, 49, 126–27
   of other pharmacy students, 92–93
   of preceptor and other health professionals, 92–93
   as two-way street, 92–93
   in work experience, 81b, 83
professional organizations
   conduct in, 53–54
   on curriculum vitae, 44, 157
   documenting participation in, 44–45
   information on, 45, 50t–51t
   involvement in, 41–54
   membership benefits of, 42–43
   networking in, 43, 119, 120–22
   online resources/opportunities, 49
   plan for participating in, 44, 46t–47t
   platform or poster presentation to, 140–41, 142f
   writing and submitting abstract to, 140
project evaluation, 71–72
project management, 65, 69–72
   action plans in, 69–70, 71t
   delegation in, 71–72
   goals and objectives in, 69–70, 71t
   meetings in, 71–72
   spreadsheet for, 71t

strategies and tactics of, 66t
proof of concept, 135
prospective study, 137
protocol, for research project, 135–39
publication, 140, 156, 174
public speaking, 156
PubMed, 174

## Q

qualifications. *See* candidates
quality assurance studies, 138
quinidine-induced torsades de pointes, 135–36

## R

RAP. *See* residency application portfolio
realistic goals, 66–67, 66t
reasonable goals, 66–67, 66t
recommendation, letters of. *See* letters of recommendation
references. *See also* letters of recommendation
 choosing, for residency application, 180–81
 on curriculum vitae, 109
reflection
 in continuous professional development, 31
 on curriculum vitae, 150–51
 self-, in service learning, 53
 in time management, 66, 68
reflective questions, in interview, 184
relevant goals, 7–10, 8b–9b
required rotations, 95
research, 80, 129–45
 altruistic reasons for, 130–31
 analysis of data from, 139
 completion of, 139
 cost and scope of, 132–33
 on curriculum vitae, 156
 definition of, 131
 design and protocol for, 135–39
 disseminating results of, 139–43
 issue/question for, 131–33, 132f, 133f
 literature search on topic, 133–34
 mentor for, 132–35, 141
 platform or poster presentation of, 140–41, 142f
 pragmatic reasons for, 130
 steps of project, 131–45, 132f
 submission of
  writing abstract for professional meeting, 140
  writing paper for journal, 141–43, 143f
Residency and Fellowship Forum (ACCP), 174–75
residency application portfolio (RAP), 159–60
residency program(s)
 academic affiliation of, 172
 accredited, 170, 178
 application process for, 15, 120, 178–92. *See also* candidates
 best fit in, 178
 characteristics of, 171–73
 competition for, 15, 149–50, 179–80
 institution/environment of, 171–72

interview for, 183–85, 189
 locating information on, 173–75
 The Match for, 150, 186–89
 nonaccredited, 170
 number of residents in, 15, 172–73
 options for, 14–15, 16t–17t, 170
 PGY1 versus PGY2, 170
 research on, 170–75
 rotations and program requirements of, 173
 selection for interview, 178–80
 thank you letters to, 185–86, 189, 192
 tips and pearls on, 179t
 training philosophy of, 173
residency program director (RPD)
 appealing CV for, 151–52
 application review and scoring by, 179–80
 goal of, 152
 interview with, 184
Residency Showcase (ASHP), 77–78, 174, 176–77
retrospective case studies, 135–36
review papers, 144–45
Rho Chi Society, 39, 48, 51t
Rosen, Kenneth, 140
rotations
 in experiential education, 95
 in residency programs, 173
rounding, interdisciplinary, 105–6, 171
RPD. *See* residency program director

## S

satisfaction, personal, 38
scheduling, 68
scheduling rotations, 95
scholarship (scholarly activities), 80, 129–45
 of application, 131
 on curriculum vitae, 156
 definition of, 131
 of discovery, 131. *See also* research
 of engagement, 131
scrambling, post-Match, 188, 188t
selection panel, 151
self-directed learning, 28–30
 in continuing education, 30–32
 definition of, 28–29
 tips for, 29–30
self-initiative, 61
self-knowledge, 2–10
self-management, 10–14, 65–72
self-reflection, 53, 150–51
self-starters, 61
servant leaders, 63
service learning, 53
*The 7 Habits of Highly Effective People* (Covey), 13
Shackleton, Ernest, 59–60
shadowing, 79–80, 122–23
skills
 constructive use of, 2
 overlap with passion, 3–10, 3f
 self-assessment of, 2–10
SMART goals, 7–10, 8b–9b, 66–67, 66t, 69

social events, 48–49, 121
social networking groups, 49, 126–27
speaking experience, 156
specific goals, 7–10, 8b–9b, 66–67, 66t
state associations, 45–48
structural frame leaders, 62
studying
   with others, 29
   for understanding, 29–30, 33
success
   aligning passion and skills in, 3
   in experiential education, 109, 110b–111b
   grades as predictor of, 34
   habits of mind and, 10, 13–14, 13b
   mentors and, 20
   mindset and, 10–14
summer internships, 78
symbolic leaders, 62–63

## T

talents
   constructive use of, 2
   overlap with passion, 3–10, 3f
   self-assessment of, 2–10
teaching activities, 80
teaching certificate program, 172
team etiquette, 105
team relationships, 100–106
tenure-track faculty, 134–35
thank you letters, 185–86, 189, 192
thinking
   critical, 93–95
   about thinking, 14
time-bound goals, 7–10, 8b–9b
time management, 39, 65–68
   matrix for, 67–68
   prioritization in, 66, 67–68
   reflection in, 66, 68
   scheduling in, 68
   SMART goals and, 66–67, 66t
   strategies and tactics of, 66t
   taking action in, 66, 68
   work experience and, 81b, 83
time-related goals, 66–67, 66t
training options, 14–15, 16t–17t, 170
training philosophy, 173
transactional leaders, 19t
transformational leaders, 19t, 63
travel costs, 178
trust, 37–38, 106

## U

understanding, studying for, 29–30
urgency, in time management matrix, 67–68

## V

VA. *See* Veterans Affairs hospitals
verapamil, and ventricular rate, 135

verbal abuse, 92
Veterans Affairs (VA) hospitals, 171–72
vocation, 3–10, 3f, 5b
   personal mission statement and, 4–7, 5b
   SMART goals and, 7–10, 8b–9b
volunteering
   on curriculum vitae, 157
   work experience through, 79–80

## W

Web-based portfolio, 36–37
Web sites, of residency programs, 174
work experience, 19, 75–87
   academic (teaching and research), 80
   advice to candidate on, 85–87, 86b
   benefits of, 75, 80–84, 81b
   career insight from, 81–82, 81b
   classroom performance enhanced by, 81, 81b
   in community pharmacies, 76–77, 78
   on curriculum vitae, 155–56
   downsides to, 83–84
   in experiential education (IPPEs and APPEs), 76–78
   finding opportunities for, 80
   in hospitals, 77, 78
   interview experience in, 81b, 84–85
   and licensure, 76, 81b, 83
   in nontraditional areas, 78
   professionalism in, 81b, 83
   relationships developed in, 81–82, 81b
   time management in, 81b, 83
   understanding gained through, 81, 81b
   variety of, 78–80
   in volunteering or shadowing, 79–80
worldview, 10. *See also* mindset

# DISCLOSURE OF POTENTIAL CONFLICTS OF INTEREST

*Consultancies:* Jerry L. Bauman (First Data Bank; McGraw-Hill; Pharmacotherapy Inc.); Bradley A. Boucher (Zymogenetics/Bristol-Myers Squibb); Janet P. Engle (Edelman; U.S. Food and Drug Administration); Curtis E. Haas (FL RX Pharmacy and Therapeutics Committee [Excellus Blue Cross/Blue Shield]; Guidepoint Global; Board of Pharmacy Specialties); Stuart T. Haines (American Association of Colleges of Pharmacy/Proctor and Gamble [spouse]; American Society of Health-System Pharmacists/ASHP Advantage); Michelle Kucera (Stormont-Vail Health Care [spouse]); Joseph Lassiter (Naturopathic Formulary Council; Oregon Patient Safety Commission; The Robertson Group); Erin M. Nystrom (American Society of Health-System Pharmacists); Beth Bryles Phillips (American Society of Health-System Pharmacists); Garrett E. Schramm (South Dakota State University Dean's Advisory Panel)

*Grants:* Janet P. Engle (Jesse Brown VA Medical Center); Dana P. Hammer (American Association of Colleges of Pharmacy; Josiah Macy Jr. Foundation); Brian Hemstreet (Astra Zeneca); Robert B. Parker (National Institutes of Health); Brandon J. Patterson (Community Pharmacy Foundation); Garrett E. Schramm (Optimer Pharmaceuticals); James E. Tisdale (American Heart Association)

*Honoraria/Speaker's Bureau:* Bradley A. Boucher (Pharmacy Learning Network; Zymogenetics); Dana P. Hammer (American College of Clinical Pharmacy); Beth Bryles Phillips (American Society of Health-System Pharmacists; McGraw-Hill); Robert E. Smith (American Association of Colleges of Pharmacy; American College of Clinical Pharmacy; North Dakota State University); James E. Tisdale (American Society of Health-System Pharmacists; California Society of Hospital Pharmacists; 4th National Conference on Drug Injury and Safe Drug Use, Beijing, China; Nevada Society of Hospital Pharmacists; Postgraduate Healthcare Education); Thomas D. Zlatic (American College of Clinical Pharmacy)

**Stock Ownership; Relationships with Companies or Vendors:** Stuart T. Haines (APhA-ASHP Partnership; Rx Instructional Systems)